40+ GUIDE TO FITNESS

40+ GUIDE TO FITNESS

DAVID STUTZ, M.D.

AND THE EDITORS OF CONSUMER REPORTS BOOKS

CONSUMER REPORTS BOOKS

A DIVISION OF CONSUMERS UNION

YONKERS, NEW YORK

To Karen

Copyright © 1994 by David Stutz

Drawings by Deborah Stutz

Published by Consumers Union of United States, Inc., Yonkers, New York 10703.

Library of Congress Cataloging-in-Publication Data

Stutz, David R.
   40+ guide to fitness / by David Stutz and the Editors of Consumer
Reports Books.
      p.   cm.
   Includes bibliographical references and index.
   ISBN 0-89043-578-2
   1. Physical fitness.   2. Middle-aged persons—Health and hygiene.
I. Consumer Reports Books.   II. Title.   III. Title: Forty plus
guide to fitness.
GV481.S77   1994
613.7—dc20   93-36375
                                               CIP

Design by GDS/Jeffrey L. Ward

First printing, February 1994

This book is printed on recycled paper.

Manufactured in the United States of America

40+ Guide to Fitness is a Consumer Reports Book published by Consumers Union, the nonprofit organization that publishes *Consumer Reports,* the monthly magazine of test reports, product Ratings, and buying guidance. Established in 1936, Consumers Union is chartered under the Not-for-Profit Corporation Law of the State of New York.
   The purposes of Consumers Union, as stated in its charter, are to provide consumers with information and counsel on consumer goods and services, to give information on all matters relating to the expenditure of the family income, and to initiate and to cooperate with individual and group efforts seeking to create and maintain decent living standards.
   Consumers Union derives its income solely from the sale of *Consumer Reports* and other publications. In addition, expenses of occasional public service efforts may be met, in part, by nonrestrictive, noncommercial contributions, grants, and fees. Consumers Union accepts no advertising or product samples and is not beholden in any way to any commercial interest. Its Ratings and reports are solely for the use of the readers of its publications. Neither the Ratings, nor the reports, nor any Consumers Union publications, including this book, may be used in advertising or for any commercial purpose. Consumers Union will take all steps open to it to prevent such uses of its material, its name, or the name of *Consumer Reports.*

Contents

Acknowledgments

I would like to acknowledge my agent, Bert Holtje, and my editors, Roz Siegel and Mark Hoffman, whose interest and support helped me transform a proposal into a completed project. I owe a debt of gratitude to the medical librarians at Sarasota Memorial Hospital, Sarasota, Florida, for their expert assistance in locating some of the materials that fleshed out the plan. Thanks are also due Ken Schields of the Sarasota Therapy Center for providing valuable input concerning rehabilitation after injury. I'm grateful to doctors Marc Grinberg, Alan Treiman, and Don Slevin, who let me pick their brains about aspects of exercise related to their medical specialties. Special recognition goes to my daughter, Deborah Stutz. She took the models we made with Humancad Mannequin Designer© software and then created the illustrations that appear in the book. The finished production would not have been possible without the valuable contributions of Rebecca Wild Baxter and Karen and Steve Feldman. Finally, thanks to my son, Aaron Stutz, who shared the Washington, D.C., Marine Corps Marathon with me, confirming the importance of my being fit after 40.

1

YOUR BODY— A WONDERFUL MACHINE

Your body is a wonderful machine, and it works best when it is used regularly. There is truth to the aphorism "Use it or lose it." As you grow older, routine physical exercise is absolutely necessary if you want to remain active, vital, and independent.

Exercise experts from the American Heart Association declare that regular, dynamic physical activity can improve cardiovascular fitness and at the same time help prevent cardiovascular disease. Other researchers point out that improving physical fitness enhances confidence and self-esteem, and increases a sense of independence at any age. The simple fact is that if you're physically active, you're healthier.

Almost 2,000 years ago, the Roman statesman Cicero wisely observed that "exercise and temperance can preserve something of our early vigor even in old age." His words are still true today.

THE BENEFITS OF EXERCISE

You can exercise in many different ways, and the beneficial effects are similar. Exercise programs include a wide range of activities that require different degrees of strength, power, skill, and endurance. Moreover, different activities expose you to varying amounts of strain on the bones, joints, muscles, and connective tissues.

The choices among activities that provide exercise are so broad and so varied that you are sure to find some appealing form of exercise. And if you engage in activities you enjoy, you're far more likely to exercise regularly.

As you get older, there are normal, predictable changes in your physical abilities. These changes may influence what you do and how long, hard, and frequently you do it. But one thing is clear: Whether you are 40 or 90, you can benefit from regular physical activity.

TABLE 1.1   CHANGES WITH AGING AND EFFECTS ON EXERCISE

	CHANGES WITH AGING	EFFECTS ON EXERCISE
MUSCLE	Gradual decrease in muscle mass between ages 20 and 50, then a more rapid drop from age 50 to 90. Despite a decrease in the total amount of muscle tissue, at least until age 70 there is no decrease in either anaerobic or aerobic potential of the muscle tissue.	Generalized loss of strength. But no matter how old you are, you still can achieve a training effect when the muscle is not yet functioning at its maximal potential, either aerobically or anaerobically.
BONE	After ages 30 to 40, 0.3 to 0.5 percent loss of bone mass per year in both men and women, increasing to 2 to 3 percent per year for women during the 6 to 10 years after menopause.	No loss of function per se, but there's a greater risk of traumatic fractures in general, and stress fractures of the vertebrae, feet, and bones of the legs—especially during impact activities.
CARTILAGE	Decreased water content and elasticity.	Greater risk of degeneration and injury, especially in weight-bearing joints such as the knees.
LIGAMENTS AND TENDONS	Decreased elasticity in ligaments and tendons.	Increased strains and sprains, especially if stretching programs and warm-up are inadequate. Decreased flexibility and reach.
NERVOUS SYSTEM	Decline in the number of nerves that serve the muscles, and a slowing in the speed of nerve impulses by 10 to 15 percent.	Decreasing reaction time, reflexes, and balance with decreasing performance in racquet sports or other "skill" sports. Increased risk of falling.
LUNGS, HEART, AND CIRCULATION	From ages 20 to 65, total heart pumping ability (cardiac output) decreases about 8 percent per decade. Steady decline in maximal heart rate and maximum oxygen consumption. Maximum air movement per breath decreases 40 to 50 percent by age 70. Cholesterol plaques (atherosclerosis) may inhibit blood supply to legs.	Overall decrease in maximum aerobic capacity, resulting in decreasing peak performance in swimming, running, cycling, and other aerobic activities. Slower recovery after aerobic activities. Greater sensitivity to extremes of heat and cold.
KIDNEYS	Gradually decreasing ability of the kidneys to filter metabolic waste products and to conserve fluid.	Increased vulnerability to extremes of heat.

Relaxation and Mental Functioning

Many regular exercisers feel calm and relaxed when they finish their workout. Walking, jogging, cycling, bench-stepping, or any repetitive activity that lasts for at least 10 minutes can induce a tranquilizing effect comparable to biofeedback or meditation. Further, psychologists who studied men and women ages 45 to 48 found that those who exercised regularly were better able to remember, solve problems, and reason than those who didn't exercise.

Mood and Sleep

Vigorous exercise induces an increase in endorphins. These natural morphinelike substances may be responsible for the mood elevation that people experience after exercise. As long as you don't exercise within three or four hours before you go to bed, aerobic activity can help you sleep more soundly. Exercising close to bedtime, however, disrupts sleep, possibly because of exercise-induced rises in body temperature that alter the usual pattern of bodily functions (circadian rhythms).

Weight Control and Exercise

A popular misconception is that exercise stimulates your appetite. In fact, a sedentary life-style interferes much more with appetite control. Unlike active people, sedentary individuals tend to eat even when they do not need the calories. Controlled studies of overweight men and women show that a regular walking or jogging program helps to restore an appropriate appetite. In other words, people who exercise tend naturally to consume only the number of calories they burn up during the course of a day.

Exercise makes a positive contribution to any weight-loss program (see Table 1.2). If you diet but do not combine exercise with your eating plan, 35 to 45 percent of the weight you lose will be lean body tissue and water, not fat. Walking briskly for 30 minutes four days a week helps you replace some of your calorie-rich fat with lean muscle tissue. This explains why overweight people who start to exercise often lose inches before they lose pounds.

Cardiac Benefits of Exercise

According to the American Heart Association, there are about 6 million Americans who have symptoms of coronary artery disease. Millions more have significant, but as yet undiagnosed, "silent" heart disease. Each year, more than 500,000 people undergo surgical procedures to open or bypass their blocked arteries. Doctors expect that in a single year, 1.5 million Americans will have heart attacks; one-third of them will die.

Researchers at the Centers for Disease Control point out that 102 million out of the 176 million Americans over age 18 are physically inactive. They note that being sedentary doubles the risk of dying from coronary artery disease, which leads to an estimated 22,000 preventable deaths in the United States every year. Older research involving male populations as varied as British bus

TABLE 1.2 CALORIES BURNED DURING EXERCISE

The number of calories you burn during any activity depends partly on your body weight (WT) and partly on the intensity of your effort.

ACTIVITY	WT 105	WT 120	WT 135	WT 150	WT 165	WT 180	WT 195	WT 210	WT 225
Bicycling 1 mile	34	38	43	48	53	58	62	67	72
Cross-country skiing, 1 mile	105	120	135	150	165	180	195	210	225
Hiking, 1 mile, 17:30 pace	85	98	110	122	134	146	159	171	183
Jogging, 1 mile	84	96	108	120	132	144	156	168	180
Swimming, 400 yards									
25 yds./min.	67	77	86	96	106	115	125	134	144
50 yds./min.	70	80	90	100	110	120	130	140	150
butterfly 50 yds./min.	79	90	101	112	123	135	146	157	168
Walking, 1 mile									
24:00 pace	50	58	65	72	79	86	94	101	108
20:00 pace	52	59	67	74	81	89	96	104	111
17:00 pace	56	64	72	80	88	96	104	112	120
15:00 pace	57	66	74	82	90	98	107	115	123
12:00 pace	69	79	89	99	109	119	129	139	148

drivers and conductors in 1966, San Francisco longshoremen in 1975, and Harvard alumni in 1978 shows that more physical activity lowers the risk of coronary artery disease. Recent research involving both male and female populations confirms the beneficial effects for women as well as men.

RISK FACTORS FOR CORONARY ARTERY DISEASE

Cigarette smoking
Hypertension
Elevated blood cholesterol
Diabetes
Decreased HDL cholesterol
Family history of heart attack under 55 years of age
Male gender
Physical inactivity
Obesity

HOW MUCH EXERCISE DO YOU NEED?

Burning up as few as 500 calories a week through exercise appears to be beneficial. A 1989 study of 10,224 men and 3,120 women by the Institute for Aerobics Research in Dallas suggests that even the modest degree of exercise you get from walking, climbing stairs, gardening, and other light leisure activities will significantly lower cardiac risk.

How Exercise Lowers Cardiac Risk

Endurance exercise performed regularly lowers blood pressure, decreases triglyceride levels in the blood, and increases the proportion of HDL or "good" cholesterol. Exercise reduces the occurrence of serious irregular heart rhythms and sudden death. It also helps to prevent blood clots in the coronary arteries, the final event that causes a heart attack.

Increased physical activity has *indirect* benefits as well. Smokers who exercise tend to smoke less. Moreover, regular activity helps you lose weight and keep it off. An exercise program helps to lower hostility, anger, and stress—precisely the traits associated with the stereotypical type-A, "coronary-prone" individual.

Exercise and the Prevention of Other Diseases

The Dallas institute's study found that people who maintain higher levels of fitness are less likely to die from various types of cancer. Moreover, a 1991 survey of 5,990 male alumni of the University of Pennsylvania showed that the incidence of diabetes declined in proportion to the amount of energy expended each week (a reduction of 6 percent for each 500 calories burned by exercise). The researchers concluded that the development of adult-onset noninsulin-dependent diabetes may be delayed by regular physical activity.

Effects of Exercise on Osteoporosis

Until the age of 30 or 35, there is a net buildup of bone mineral. But around age 40, both men and women begin to experience a loss of bone mineral. Because of declining estrogen levels, women go through a period of more rapid bone loss starting at menopause and continuing for 10 years or more. These changes contribute to the development of osteoporosis—the major cause of an estimated 250,000 hip fractures, 500,000 spine fractures, and 240,000 wrist fractures each year in the United States. Most of these injuries involve women.

Regular physical activity is important for maintaining the structural integrity of your bones as you get older. The combination of exercise and calcium supplementation can slow down, prevent, and even reverse bone-mineral loss in women. Furthermore, exercise increases the protective effects of estrogen replacement therapy for women whose bone density may already be low. In short, there are so many benefits and so many different kinds of exercise that are easy, accessible, inexpensive, and safe that it is hard to find a reason *not* to exercise.

Before choosing the exercise or sport that is best for you, it is helpful to learn more about how physical exertion affects your body.

THE BASIC PHYSIOLOGY OF EXERCISE

No matter how intense or casual your exercise program, any physical activity should involve

- muscles, tendons, bones, and ligaments that move and bear the physical stresses of activity
- energy production for muscle contraction
- efficient removal of the waste products that exercise generates

The Biomechanics of Exercise

Tendons, bones, cartilage, and ligaments are the physical linkages that turn muscle contractions into body movements. The forces that these structures sustain during exercise are enormous. For example, when you run, you hit the ground with an impact of two and one-half to three times your body weight with each stride. If you weigh 150 pounds, this means absorbing roughly 220 tons of force per mile! With many activities, you also add the stresses of repeated wear and tear caused by throwing, kicking, and moving from side to side.

High-impact and low-impact activity. As you hit the ground, forces are transmitted up through the bones, cartilage, and ligaments. Each repeated movement multiplies the impact on the feet, knees, hips, and back. Potentially, this is a problem because repeated impact may bring on joint and cartilage damage, stress fractures in the feet and legs, and compression fractures in the mid and lower spine.

Activities that are considered *high-impact* include jogging and running, basketball, volleyball, and some aerobics. *Low-impact* activities include walking, cycling, swimming, rowing, cross-country skiing, sailing, some fishing, and some aerobics.

Energy Production and Muscle Contraction

Metabolic chemical reactions that produce energy are necessary for muscles to contract. The chemical medium that actually provides the energy for muscle contraction is a compound called adenosine triphosphate (ATP). Muscles can store only a small amount of ATP, and that supply is depleted after only 25 seconds of maximal effort. Consequently, to sustain activity beyond an initial surge, you have to continue to regenerate your supply of ATP.

In your muscles, ATP is produced by metabolic reactions that are either *anaerobic* (do not use oxygen) or *aerobic* (require oxygen). Anaerobic metabolism provides a large amount of energy quickly, so it is most important when you are beginning your activity or when you need a surge of power. However, the fuel for anaerobic metabolism is limited to a simple carbohydrate, glucose, which is stored in muscles as glycogen. The supply is exhausted after two or three minutes of maximal exercise. In the process of generating energy, anaerobic reactions produce relatively large amounts of waste products, such as lactic acid.

In contrast, aerobic energy production produces ATP more slowly but much more efficiently. Aerobic metabolism utilizes a wide range of fuels, and aerobic reactions burn those fuels more completely. Unlike anaerobic ATP production, aerobic energy production is able to sustain activity for hours at a time, and the fuel supply for aerobic metabolism is essentially limitless.

Most exercises and athletic activities require a combination of both aerobic and anaerobic energy production. However, the terms *aerobic* and *anaerobic* are also used to describe activities that are powered primarily by one type of metabolism or the other. Typically, aerobic exercise involves near-continuous activity such as walking, jogging, bicycling, swimming, and cross-country skiing. Anaerobic exercise incorporates sudden or repeated bursts of activity, characteristic of sprinting, weight training, and downhill skiing. Generally, the terms *aerobic exercise, sustained activity, dynamic exercise,* and *endurance training* are used interchangeably. The terms *anaerobic activity, resistance exercise, strength training,* and *nonsustained activity* are used synonymously. Table 1.3 lists 25 activities, from most aerobic to least aerobic.

Heart, Lung, and Circulatory Responses

Predictable changes take place in your heart, lungs, and blood vessels when you exercise. Your heart beats more rapidly, accelerating from roughly 60 beats per minute at rest to as many as 180 or more during sustained activity. This may increase the amount of blood pumped per minute (your cardiac output) by as much as 500 percent. The changes in lung function are even more dramatic, with the amount of air going in and out of the lungs increasing up to twentyfold after exercise.

TABLE 1.3   TWENTY-FIVE EXERCISE ACTIVITIES, FROM MOST AEROBIC TO LEAST AEROBIC

Every activity is partly aerobic and partly anaerobic. The activities at the top of the list are the most aerobic because they require the most continuous and steady effort and therefore use the greatest amount of oxygen during activity.

1. Jogging and running	10. Martial arts	18. Alpine skiing
2. Cross-country skiing	11. Basketball	19. Weight training
3. Rowing and canoeing	12. Roller skating	20. Horseback riding
4. Swimming	13. Ice skating	21. Baseball
5. Bicycling	14. Tennis	22. Fishing
6. Aerobic dance	15. Volleyball	23. Golf
7. Hiking and climbing	16. Walking	24. Bowling
8. Soccer	17. Football	25. Sailing
9. Racquetball and squash		

Your arteries and veins respond to exercise by sending as much as 85 percent of your blood to the muscles (at the expense of internal organs such as the intestinal tract and the kidneys). As heart pumping increases, systolic blood pressure, which is normally less than 130 millimeters of mercury (mm Hg) at rest, approaches 180 to 200 mm Hg. Diastolic pressure usually stays the same or falls because the arteries open wider (dilate) to supply more blood to the working muscles. However, during sustained anaerobic activity such as weight lifting or cycling up a steep hill, there is less dilation of the arteries. Systolic pressure may exceed 220, and diastolic pressure may exceed 150 for as long as several minutes. This dramatic rise is generally safe for people whose blood pressure is normal and who have no heart or vascular disease.

Gastrointestinal and Urinary Systems

The gastrointestinal and urinary systems "shut off" during sustained activity because most of the blood flow is diverted to the muscles. During vigorous exercise, any food in the stomach tends to sit there. This explains why you feel bloated and full if you exercise too soon after you eat. The decrease in blood flow to the kidneys also means that you don't usually need to urinate while you are exercising.

Metabolic Waste Removal

The two major metabolic waste products that must be removed from the muscles during exercise are lactic acid and heat. Lactic acid is produced when glucose is metabolized to generate ATP during anaerobic metabolism. As lactic acid accumulates, you may feel burning in the muscles, pain, or fatigue. Lactic acid continues to build up as you exercise anaerobically. After you slow down, most of it is "recycled" metabolically as fuel for aerobic reactions.

The buildup of heat is much more problematic, because if your body temperature gets too high, you may collapse and even die. When you run, you generate 15 to 18 times more heat than you do at rest. If this heat were simply allowed to build up, your body temperature would rise 1.8°F (1°C) every five minutes, leading to collapse within about 30 minutes. Fortunately, our bodies have several very efficient mechanisms to remove (excrete) the heat generated during exercise.

NUTRITIONAL ASPECTS OF EXERCISE

There is probably more myth and misunderstanding in the area of athletic diet and nutrition than in almost any other topic related to exercise. To meet your own nutritional and energy needs, it's helpful to understand how different food substances are metabolized.

The Role of Carbohydrates

Carbohydrate molecules, which are either sugars or strings of sugars connected together, are found in refined and unrefined sweets as well as in grains and most fruits and vegetables. Carbohydrates produce 116 calories per ounce (4.1 calories of energy per gram), and they're the cleanest-burning fuel used by your muscles: They give off only carbon dioxide and water when completely burned for energy. A small amount of carbohydrate in the form of glycogen is stored in the muscles themselves. This energy reserve provides fuel for anaerobic reactions, and it's vital for preventing muscle fatigue during aerobic endurance activities. By eating carbohydrate-rich foods before exercise, you build up crucial glycogen stores in the muscles—a process known as *carbohydrate loading*. For this reason, many marathon runners eat pasta exclusively the night before a run.

Protein

Protein, which is composed of nitrogen-containing amino acids, is found in meats of all kinds, in most nuts and seeds, and in dairy products, egg whites, and vegetables such as legumes. Although you need dietary protein to build and repair muscle, once you have taken in enough to satisfy your body's maintenance needs, any remaining protein is transformed into sugar. If that sugar is not immediately utilized for energy production, the calories are stored as fat. When pure protein is completely metabolized, it yields 122 calories per ounce (4.3 calories per gram), almost the same number as carbohydrates. However, protein doesn't burn as cleanly as carbohydrate, because it leaves nitrogen waste products. This nitrogen is transformed into urea that is eliminated by the kidneys, unavoidably carrying water out of the body.

You probably don't need to eat extra protein just because you're exercising. Even if you do intensive weight training, your protein needs will be satisfied by a normal diet. Protein supplements aren't necessary for building muscle bulk. In fact, protein requirements for weight lifters are generally less than those for endurance athletes, who derive about 10 percent of their energy from protein used as a fuel source during strenuous and aerobic exercise.

Fat

Fat, composed almost entirely of carbon and hydrogen, is the most concentrated fuel in the body. Fat generates 264 calories per ounce (9.3 calories per gram), and, all things being equal, you would have to burn off 4,224 calories to lose one pound of fat. (You have to metabolize only 1,920 calories in order to burn up one pound of protein or carbohydrate.) Whether you eat carbohydrates, proteins, or fats, all three must be immediately utilized for fuel or they are stored in the body as fat tissue.

Since fat constitutes the largest reservoir of energy, it's the body's preferred source of fuel during sustained aerobic activity. It also provides the majority of the calories used during aerobic activities such as jogging, cycling, swimming, or walking, once you've settled into a comfortable pace. But since any unused carbohydrates or proteins are stored as fat, fat consumption itself should be kept to a minimum.

Vitamins and Minerals

A healthful diet that is sufficient to meet your caloric needs will also be adequate to satisfy your overall requirements for vitamins and minerals. There is no evidence that supplementary vitamins improve an athlete's performance. Although most vitamins appear to have little potential for harm, avoid large supplemental doses of vitamins A and D because of the toxic effects that have been reported with excessive intake.

Iron and calcium are another matter. Following impact sports such as karate or intensive jogging, your requirements for iron may increase as a result of muscle damage and subsequent iron loss in the urine. Women with heavy menstrual bleeding may require additional iron, and calcium supplements are advisable for women to help prevent osteoporosis.

In general, however, a diet low in fat, with generous portions of fruits and vegetables, should be sufficient for an exercise program. Supplementary vitamins, minerals, or other nutrients are not needed.

2
GETTING STRONGER
WITH EXERCISE

Regular exercise is not only good for your *health*—it's good for your *life*. Weakness and physical inactivity are not an automatic part of the aging process. Rather, inactive life-style is the primary cause of muscle weakness, and regular exercise can slow and even reverse much of the expected decline in exercise capacity and muscle strength that occurs as we get older. Even if you haven't been active for years, you can still make significant gains in muscle strength and exercise endurance. The choice is up to you.

THE TRAINING EFFECT

Anyone who exercises knows that the more you do, the easier it becomes. This phenomenon of building strength, endurance, and skill is called the *training effect*. The two main principles that govern the training effect are (1) specificity and (2) overload and reinforcement. *Specificity* means that you develop only what you actually use; *overload and reinforcement* refer to the fact that you achieve your improvement only if you do more work than you are accustomed to doing, and that you maintain your improvement only if you continue your activities.

Training the Muscles

When you lift, pull, or push at close to your maximal capacity, you develop stronger and generally larger muscles. Moreover, the connecting tendons and ligaments become stronger with prudent regular training. This is as true for 90-year-olds as it is for teenagers, and it applies both to men and to women. During the first three weeks of weight training, most of the increase in muscle strength comes from a more efficient interaction between the nerves and the muscle fibers. Increases in real muscle bulk may take as long as three to five weeks. Because of hormonal differences, the effects are more pronounced in men than in women.

As you exert yourself aerobically or anaerobically, you also increase your muscles' endurance—

it takes longer for them to become fatigued. Aerobic physical activity improves muscle energy production by actually increasing the quantity of aerobic metabolic enzymes. This increase in enzymes, which may be as much as 100 percent, allows muscles to produce ATP much more easily. Anaerobic exercise improves muscle endurance in a different way by increasing the amount of ATP that is stored in the muscle tissue.

Increasing muscle strength and endurance doesn't necessarily improve your performance in "skill" sports such as golf, tennis, or baseball. These activities rely more on timing and coordination than on strength. When you train for these sports, you generally focus on practicing the skills themselves. However, for any level of skill, exercise training to increase strength and flexibility gives you extra endurance and produces less muscle fatigue, allowing you to perform better and longer.

Training the Heart and Circulation

Part of the improvement in stamina and strength, especially with aerobic activities, results from more efficiency in the heart and circulation. Your heart's ability to pump blood can actually double with endurance training. More of the blood will be directed to the working muscles because the stimulation of muscle activity makes these arteries open up (dilate). The same arterial dilation tends to lower systolic and diastolic blood pressure, and the effects continue even when you're not exercising. All of these changes mean that your muscles receive more oxygen, allowing them to work for longer periods of time. And better performance of the heart and circulatory system means that you won't get out of breath as easily.

You will see considerable improvement in only several weeks if you begin exercising just below the threshold of breathlessness for 20-minute sessions two or three times a week. Those people who are in the poorest physical shape to begin with—and who have the most to gain—are the very people who show the most rapid improvement in the pumping efficiency of the heart, about a 20 percent increase in pumping capacity in only a few weeks. However, if you're already functioning at a high level of fitness, your workouts will have to be even more intensive if you want to progress further.

Maintaining the Training Effect

In general, once you have built up aerobic and anaerobic strength and endurance, it takes much less of an effort to *maintain* it than it did to develop it in the first place. For example, if you have worked out vigorously four or five times per week for several months, you can reduce the frequency and duration of your workouts by as much as two-thirds and still keep nearly the same level of aerobic fitness—as long as you don't reduce the *intensity* of each workout.

The more fit you are when you cut back on your exercise schedule, the easier it is for you to maintain a high level of strength and fitness. When elite athletes completely stop an ongoing, high-intensity weight-lifting program, it takes 12 weeks to lose roughly 70 percent of the strength they had previously gained. However, by continuing just one high-intensity workout per week, these athletes can maintain most of their strength almost indefinitely. The average regular exerciser may lose strength more rapidly than this, and the loss of strength with inactivity is even more pronounced for beginning exercisers. Beginners may gain muscle strength and endurance more quickly, but they also lose the training effects more rapidly once they stop working out.

Cross-Training

Cross-training is a simple concept. By varying the types of activities you do, you exercise different parts of your body on different days. In this way, you build up cardiovascular fitness while minimizing the risks of impact and overuse injury. For example, jogging relies on the muscles in the back of the thighs, bicycling primarily uses the muscles in the front of the thighs, and swimming engages the legs, arms, and shoulders. By alternating these activities, you will enhance your aerobic stamina while giving specific muscle groups time to rest and recover from exertion. Cross-training has become so popular that many formerly dedicated joggers now take part in triathlons (races that combine swimming, cycling, and running).

Combining Programs for Aerobic and Strength Training

Almost all forms of exercise are partly aerobic and partly anaerobic. When you combine both endurance and strength training programs, you improve your overall exercise capability as well as your performance in specific activities. For example, weight training to strengthen the arms, shoulders, and upper chest makes any lifting, pulling, or pushing easier to do. Rowers obviously benefit, but so do joggers, who experience less arm fatigue during long-distance runs. Likewise, by increasing aerobic endurance with a jogging program, it is possible for equestrians, climbers, and sailors to push harder and longer before becoming short of breath. If your goal is to develop both aerobic endurance and muscle strength, you can do the appropriate exercises either during a single session or on different days. Some people do weight training and the treadmill on the same day, while others focus on one activity or another during an entire session.

THE BIORHYTHMS OF EXERCISE

Influences both inside and outside your body affect your exercise capability and performance. Your internal environment is constantly changing, often in ways that are predictable. These daily changes in the body's internal function are known as *circadian rhythms,* and each person's rhythms generally follow the same overall pattern on most days. Because circadian rhythms influence a variety of physiological functions, the body's ability to respond to the demands of physical activity may also change throughout the day.

The environment outside of your body also affects your ability to perform effectively and safely. Temperature, humidity, air quality, altitude, and physical terrain may impose unique demands on your body. When you understand how your body changes throughout the day and how the environment outside your body influences the physiological response to exercise, you will be able to enhance not only your exercise performance but also your ability to avoid injury.

Circadian Rhythms

Your sleep pattern, level of alertness, basal metabolism, body temperature, heart rate, blood pressure, hormonal outputs, and even the clotting ability of the blood all vary throughout the day. Most people find that their sports performance is at its best in the early afternoon, not the early morning. That's the time when body temperature, alertness, strength, and flexibility are usually at their peak and when resting heart rate, blood pressure, and morning surge in stress hormones are generally lower. Naturally, there are variations from person to person. "Morning people" tend to get up earlier and are more alert in the earlier hours of the day, whereas "night people" generally perform better in the later morning and afternoon.

Circadian rhythms may also play a role in coronary artery disease. It has long been observed that heart attacks and sudden deaths occur more frequently between 7 and 11 A.M. Not only is blood pressure lower in the early morning, but the blood-clotting platelet cells are stickier at that time as well. In addition, the blood vessels, including those in the heart, are more likely to constrict in the early morning as opposed to later in the day. However, people with coronary artery disease who exercise regularly have a lower risk of early-morning heart attacks. Moreover, in cardiac rehab programs exercising during the morning hours appears to be just as safe as exercising at other times during the day.

Female Rhythms

Most women below age 50 experience a menstrual cycle of 20 to 30 days. Intense physical training, such as marathon running and competitive gymnastics, may shorten the menstrual cycle or eliminate periods altogether. But in most cases, exercise has no effect on either the length or nature of the menstrual flow.

Women may or may not notice any effects of their hormonal cycle on exercise capacity or performance. Some female athletes do feel that their athletic performance suffers during certain phases of their menstrual cycle. Yet, a study done in 1991 at Florida State University concluded that for activity of a relatively short duration (sprint and middle-distance swimming, strength training), the cycle phase did not influence performance.

THE EFFECTS OF ENVIRONMENT ON EXERCISE

Environmental factors such as temperature, humidity, altitude, air quality, and terrain all influence your performance and your safety when you exercise. But you can adapt to a wide range of environmental conditions, and this ability to adapt to new or extreme situations is enhanced if you are physically fit.

Heat

Metabolic activity generates heat, and during intense exercise the heat production in contracting muscles can increase fifteen- to twentyfold. With vigorous activity, the rapid rise in your body temperature must be countered by very efficient heat-removal mechanisms.

One of the main factors that affect how well you are able to get rid of body heat is the temperature around you. Heat is removed from the body either by convection (from air passing over your skin), by direct radiation into cooler surroundings, or by the evaporation of sweat on your body's surface. As breezes die down and the air around you becomes warmer, convection and radiation are less effective. By the time the air temperature rises to 85° or 90°F, the only effective way to cool your body is through the evaporation of sweat. The situation is worse if the relative humidity is high, because your body's cooling by evaporation is much less efficient.

If all of your perspiration were to evaporate completely, each quart of sweat would dispose of approximately 580 calories of heat—about what your muscles produce during a 40-minute jog at a pace of 9½ minutes per mile. Unfortunately, as the humidity rises, evaporation of sweat is incomplete. As more drips off your skin, less of it contributes to cooling despite the loss of fluid. Fortunately, after you have exercised in hot and humid conditions, your body learns how to remove heat more effectively. Within 14 days of starting training, you will have reached 90 percent of your maximum heat-removal efficiency.

When you exercise, you will not feel thirsty until you have lost 2 percent of your weight in fluid (between one and two quarts of water). You can prevent difficulties by being well hydrated. Make sure your urine is light in color before you start to exercise, then drink at least one quart of water per hour during exercise in hot weather.

When you dress for exercise in the heat, you need to shield yourself from solar radiation. At the same time, you have to allow the heat you generate to escape. Light, loose, well-ventilated clothing, as well as hats and visors, provide the most comfort and protection.

Cold

Generally, exercise in the cold poses fewer problems than exercise in hot weather. Nevertheless, any part of your body that is poorly insulated or overexposed can suffer freezing damage. There are well-documented reports of frostbite involving the fingers, toes, nose, ears, and even the unexposed penis. Cold, dry air may also irritate the respiratory passages. This is more likely to happen during intense aerobic activity, when you have to breathe through your mouth, and the irritation may bring on asthma and bronchitis. For cardiac patients, the strain of exercising in the cold against the wind may cause chest pain (angina).

In cold weather, your clothing should insulate you from excessive heat loss, protect exposed areas of your body (hands, feet, head, face, and ears) from the cold and wind, and still allow you as much freedom of movement as possible. Dress in layers of relatively light clothing that will keep the wind out but still allow moisture to escape. Zippered parkas, sweat pants, and other similar garments may be either removed or opened as you heat up; they can be replaced or closed as you cool down. It's important to prepare not only for activity (when you're generating heat) but also for those periods when you slow down or stop. You will then need more insulation to conserve body heat.

Altitude

At an elevation of 8,000 feet (2,560) meters, there is only 74 percent as much oxygen in the air as there is at sea level. Under these conditions the blood oxygen concentration is reduced by 36 percent, but the body tissues adapt by extracting oxygen more efficiently from the blood. Practically speaking, few people experience any difficulty when they are at altitudes below 6,500 feet (2,000 meters). Even when you're at elevations between 6,500 and 8,000 feet, you should notice only moderately reduced aerobic stamina and possibly more labored breathing during normal activities.

Within several days of being at high altitudes, most people begin to adapt to the lower oxygen concentrations. Respiratory processes become much more efficient at a higher altitude. Many elite endurance athletes capitalize on this fact by exercising at high altitudes in order to improve their heart and lung capacity.

If you're already in good aerobic condition, you should be able to adapt quickly to higher altitudes. Generally, there's little risk in exercising at such altitudes as long as you are otherwise healthy. This was emphasized by a 1990 study in Vail, Colorado, of 100 men age 40 to 70 who skied at elevations as high as 11,250 feet (3,400 meters). These men suffered no heart or lung problems. However, if you have decreased lung capacity because of emphysema or some other lung condition, or if you have coronary artery disease, the lower level of circulating oxygen will reduce your ability to be active. This is important to consider when planning for vacation and travel.

Air Quality and Pollution

Air quality presents a special problem for exercisers. Increased levels of carbon monoxide from industrial pollution and automobile exhaust not only affect your exercise performance but also magnify the risks for people with coronary artery disease. Breathing carbon monoxide decreases the amount of oxygen that can be transported by the blood to your body's tissues. Ordinarily, this doesn't bother healthy people, but it can make a difference for heart patients. When cardiac patients are exposed to concentrations of carbon monoxide that are encountered frequently (similar to levels from cigarette smoking, driving in tunnels, stop-and-go freeway traffic, or heavy air pollution), they are much more likely to develop electrocardiographic signs of cardiac strain, angina (chest pain), and abnormalities in their heart rhythm. This occurs both with exercise and at rest.

When you breathe more deeply and rapidly (as during physical activity), you tend to concentrate carbon monoxide in the blood. This is a concern for people who jog or bicycle along the side of the road or on heavily traveled roads. Under these circumstances, almost everyone will have a transient decrease in exercise capacity.

Terrain

You may not give much thought to the surface on which you exercise, but it can affect both your comfort and performance. Harder and smoother surfaces offer less resistance to forward motion for bicyclists and runners. But for runners and joggers, harder surfaces also mean greater impact. If your activity requires swift turns or changes in direction, surfaces that are soft or slippery can be dangerous because they inhibit your traction and side-to-side stability. This may lead to sprains, pulls, and falls. Even when traction isn't a problem, walking or jogging on sloping surfaces at the edge of a road creates uneven stresses on the ankles, hips, and back.

Hills also cause difficulties, especially when you are descending. Walking or running uphill is excellent training, and the natural braking effect of gravity prevents excessive impact and falls. But when you run or walk down a steep hill, you tend to accelerate. The pull of gravity makes it much more difficult to resist those forces that cause injuries. Furthermore, if you're cycling, roller skating, or roller-blading, there's an increased chance of losing control, falling, and suffering potentially serious injury.

THE SAFETY OF REGULAR EXERCISE

From a cardiac standpoint and from an orthopedic point of view, regular exercise is generally safe, despite the occasional, well-publicized reports of sudden death.

Heart Attack and Sudden Death

Everyone's risk for cardiac arrest is slightly increased during vigorous exercise, but the risk is still very small. In 1982 a survey of the general population at 48 YMCAs and Jewish Community Centers pointed out that during 33,726,000 hours of exercise, there was only one nonfatal heart attack or cardiac arrest per 887,526 hours of participation. Moreover, only one death is reported for each 1,124,200 hours of activity. The American College of Sports Medicine estimates that only one presumably healthy man in 20,000 will suffer cardiac arrest during vigorous activity such as racquetball or jogging. Studies performed in Helsinki and Seattle show the same thing: If you're physically fit, your risk for cardiac arrest and sudden death is lower not only during the activity itself, but also through the rest of the day.

There may be an exceedingly low risk of heart attack and sudden death for apparently healthy people during vigorous exercise, yet the same is true for the higher-risk individuals who participate in supervised cardiac rehabilitation classes. In 1986, in an extensive review of 167 outpatient cardiac rehabilitation programs, it was found that among 51,303 patients who exercised 2,351,916 hours, there was only one heart attack or cardiac arrest per 81,101 patient hours of exercise and only one fatality per 783,972 hours of exercise.

Injury

Sooner or later, anyone who is active is bound to experience some type of injury. Usually, injuries are minor and heal on their own. As you increase the intensity, duration, and impact of your exercise, you also increase the frequency and the severity of strains, sprains, abrasions, tears, and even fractures. Moreover, for any level of activity, the likelihood of injury tends to increase as you get older. Fortunately, the chances of tendon, ligament, muscle, bone, or joint injuries can be minimized if you select your activities carefully and plan your schedule judiciously.

The benefits of exercise far outweigh the risks. Beyond age 40, you possess significant exercise potential. You can improve both your physical conditioning and emotional well-being. With proper equipment and a sensible regimen, you can exercise effectively and safely.

3

CHOOSING YOUR ACTIVITIES AND GETTING STARTED

People exercise for a variety of reasons. You may have a general goal, such as lowering daily stress, or you may have the very specific objective of strengthening your leg muscles for an upcoming ski trip. When you understand what you can achieve with a variety of recreational activities, you can meet a wide range of objectives. These include lowering your risk of heart attack, controlling your body weight, improving your appearance, and increasing your muscle strength.

ASSESSING THE RISKS OF EXERCISE

Before starting any exercise program, the question you should ask is, "Can I start right away, or do I need a professional medical assessment first?" Many people are concerned about the risk of having a heart attack or dying suddenly during exercise. But the life-threatening aspects have to be put in perspective. Although some sports are inherently more dangerous than others, the likelihood of an injury may depend less on what activity you do than on *how* you do it.

Cardiac Risk

The American College of Sports Medicine's *Guidelines for Exercise Testing and Prescription* divides people into three groups:

- apparently healthy people
- individuals at higher risk
- people with *known* disease

Take the test in Table 3.1 to determine whether you're at low risk or high risk for heart problems that can occur with exercise. Some of the questions presuppose that you've had a fairly recent medical checkup and that you know your blood pressure and cholesterol readings.

TABLE 3.1 DETERMINING YOUR RISK LEVEL FOR GETTING STARTED*

MAJOR CORONARY RISK FACTORS
(Mark 5 points for each risk factor that applies to you.)

1. Diagnosed hypertension with blood pressure reading ≥160/90 on at least two occasions, or on high blood pressure medication _____

2. Cholesterol ≥240 _____

3. Cigarette smoker (any amount) _____

4. Family history of coronary disease in parents or siblings before age 55 _____

AGE AND SEX
(Mark 5 points for each risk factor that applies to you.)

Male over 40 years old
Female over 50 years old _____

SYMPTOMS SUGGESTING HEART, LUNG, OR METABOLIC DISEASE
(Mark 10 points for each risk factor that applies to you.)

1. Chest, jaw, or arm pain or discomfort with physical activity, but relieved by rest _____

2. Unaccustomed shortness of breath, or shortness of breath with mild exertion _____

3. Dizziness or fainting _____

4. Shortness of breath lying down or during the night _____

5. Pain in the leg or calf during walking that is relieved by rest _____

6. Palpitations, rapid heartbeat, or known heart murmur _____

7. Swelling of the ankles _____

8. Known diabetes, whether or not requiring insulin _____

INDICATE THE INTENSITY OF EXERCISE YOU ARE PLANNING TO DO

1. *Moderate*—within your current capability so that you can sustain it comfortably for as long as 60 minutes. You plan to progress gradually (e.g., with a walking program or increasing what you are doing already). *Give yourself 0 points.* _____

2. *Vigorous*—a level of activity you have not already been doing. When you try it, your heart will beat faster and your breathing will be harder. This level of activity usually cannot be sustained by a sedentary person for more than 15 or 20 minutes (e.g., jogging). *Give yourself 5 points.* _____

TOTAL POINTS _____

If your TOTAL is 5 points or less, exercise testing prior to getting started is optional.
If your TOTAL is 10 points or more, consult your physician regarding exercise testing.

*Based on criteria developed by the American College of Sports Medicine and the American Heart Association.

Apparently healthy people. Exercise is very safe for people who are apparently healthy. In studies of large populations of healthy adults who engage in vigorous physical activity, only one death occurs each year for every 15,000 to 20,000 participants. Even sedentary adults who are apparently healthy can begin moderate exercise such as brisk walking, so long as they're alert to the development of any unusual signs and symptoms.

But what about starting more vigorous exercise that causes a significant rise in breathing and pulse rate? According to the American College of Sports Medicine guidelines, if you're an apparently healthy but untrained man over age 40 or an untrained woman over 50, it's advisable to have a medical examination and possibly a stress test before you start an exercise program.

Individuals at higher risk.   When you begin any activity program without having a medical evaluation, start to exercise gradually and in a noncompetitive environment. If you haven't experienced any of the symptoms that suggest the presence of cardiopulmonary (heart and lung) disease, diabetes, thyroid problems, kidney disease, or liver disease, formal stress testing and a special medical examination may not be necessary. *If you have two or more coronary risk factors, the American College of Sports Medicine recommends that you consult your physician about having an exercise stress test before you begin any exercise program.* The same holds true if you have symptoms suggesting the possibility of cardiopulmonary disease, diabetes, kidney disease, or thyroid disease.

People with known disease.   *If you have already been diagnosed with any of the conditions cited above, consult a physician before starting any exercise program.* A medical assessment will help you select the safest and most beneficial type of activity. At the same time, a medical consultation will help you identify potential dangers related to medications, diet, and the intensity and timing of your exercise program. As an added bonus, a stress test will measure your baseline functional capacity and serve as a standard for comparing your progress later on.

Exercise Testing (Stress Test)

There are two major reasons for undergoing exercise testing:

1. To assess your level of aerobic fitness
2. To determine the likelihood of underlying cardiac disease

The most common method of exercise testing involves the use of a treadmill. In one common protocol (Bruce Protocol), every three minutes, the speed and slope of the treadmill increase. If walking is a problem, then a stationary bicycle is used instead of the treadmill. To assess cardiac risk, exercise testing includes EKG and blood pressure monitoring, possibly combined with special imaging, to analyze how well blood flows to the heart muscle (see Table 3.2).

Some people may be unaware that they have heart disease. Moreover, there's no practical way to detect everyone who has coronary artery blockage, even when the blockage may be serious enough to cause a heart attack.

Unfortunately, exercise testing is far from perfect for identifying symptomless people who may have coronary artery disease. When exercise testing is done on people who are younger or appear healthy, positive results (when they occur) are particularly unreliable.

It is an entirely different story when exercise stress testing is performed on people who are at higher risk—people who have had a heart attack in the past; those who have typical angina symptoms, which include chest pain or pressure; and individuals who have multiple risk factors for coronary artery disease. The reliability of diagnostic exercise testing improves as you get older, simply because coronary artery disease (with or without symptoms) becomes more and more prevalent with increasing age.

TABLE 3.2 EXERCISE STRESS TEST AND COMPARABLE ACTIVITIES

BRUCE PROTOCOL

Many physicians use the Bruce Protocol. Every three minutes, you proceed to the next stage, where the treadmill goes faster and the grade increases. Exercise continues until either symptoms of angina occur, you have achieved at least 85 percent of your maximal predicted heart rate, or you are exhausted. The amount of work you do in each of the stages of exercise can be compared to the amount of effort you expend during typical occupational and recreational activities.

STAGE	MPH	GRADE	RECREATIONAL ACTIVITY	OCCUPATIONAL ACTIVITY
I	1.7	10%	Walking 3.5 mph (17:30 min/mile) Cycling 8 mph Table tennis Golf (carrying clubs) Tennis doubles Calisthenics	Painting, masonry Paperhanging Light carpentry Raking leaves Hoeing
II	2.5	12%	Walking 5 mph (12:00 min/mile) Cycling 11 mph Tennis singles Cross-country skiing 2.5 mph Waterskiing Square dancing	Shoveling 10 lbs 10 times per min Splitting wood Snow shoveling Hand lawn-mowing
III	3.4	14%	Running 5.5 mph (11:00 min/mile) Cycling 13 mph Cross-country skiing 4 mph Squash or racquetball—social Handball—social Basketball—vigorous	Shoveling 14 lbs 10 times per min
IV	4.2	16%	Running 7 mph (8:35 min/mile) Basketball, fast-break Cross-country skiing 6 mph Racquetball or squash—competitive Rowing—vigorous Soccer—competitive	
V	5.0	18%	Running 8.5 mph (7:00 min/mile) Cross-country skiing 8 mph	

SETTING YOUR GOALS

There are dozens of reasons for doing one activity or another, but for the most part it boils down to

- enhancing aerobic endurance
- controlling weight
- building and toning muscles
- reducing stress, relieving tension, and having fun

Your reasons for exercising may change from one day to the next, but that doesn't mean you need to alter your activities. For instance, you may run hard primarily to build up your aerobic capacity; you may also relieve tension by doing a slow easy run. For you, running may be just as relaxing as fishing or leisure sailing is for someone else. Table 3.3 details the extent to which the 25 activities listed in chapter 1 can satisfy the above objectives. This information provides you with a starting point from which you can make your activity selections.

Building Aerobic Endurance

If your goal is to build up your aerobic capacity, then you need to focus on those activities that require the repetitive use of your muscles, especially the large muscles of the legs. Improving your

TABLE 3.3   TWENTY-FIVE ACTIVITIES AND THE GOALS OF EXERCISE

ACTIVITY	AEROBIC TRAINING	WEIGHT CONTROL[1]	MUSCLE TRAINING[2]	STRESS REDUCTION
Aerobic dance	Very good	Very good	Poor	Very good
Alpine skiing	Fair	Poor	Good	Good
Baseball	Fair	Poor	Fair	Fair
Basketball	Very good	Good	Fair	Good
Bicycling	Excellent	Excellent	Good	Excellent
Bowling	Poor	Poor	Fair	Good
Cross-country skiing	Excellent	Excellent	Fair	Excellent
Fishing	Poor	Poor	Fair	Very Good
Football	Good	Fair	Fair	Good
Golf	Poor	Poor	Poor	Good
Hiking and climbing	Very good	Very good	Fair	Very good
Horseback riding	Fair	Fair	Fair	Good
Ice skating	Good	Fair	Fair	Good
Jogging and running	Excellent	Excellent	Fair	Excellent
Martial arts	Very good	Very good	Very good	Good
Racquetball and squash	Very good	Very good	Fair	Good
Roller skating	Good	Fair	Fair	Good
Rowing and canoeing	Excellent	Excellent	Very good	Excellent
Sailing	Poor	Poor	Fair	Excellent
Soccer	Very good	Very good	Fair	Good
Swimming	Excellent	Very good	Good	Very good
Tennis	Good	Good	Poor	Good
Volleyball	Good	Good	Fair	Good
Walking	Good	Very good	Poor	Excellent
Weight training	Fair	Good	Excellent	Good

[1]Largely dependent on the duration of activity
[2]Largely dependent on the intensity of effort

level of aerobic fitness enables you to be more active for a longer period of time—at work, at home, or while engaging in leisure activity. Ideal choices for aerobic training and fitness include walking, hiking, jogging, stair climbing, dancing, rope skipping, rowing, skating, swimming, cycling, cross-country skiing, and endurance games such as basketball and soccer.

Frequency of exercise.   The American College of Sports Medicine recommends performing an aerobic activity at least three times a week for at least 20 minutes per session. Exercising less than twice a week produces little meaningful improvement. When your workouts are more frequent than three times a week, the gain in aerobic fitness begins to level off. Once you reach five workouts per week, additional exercise will provide essentially no further aerobic benefit.

Intensity and duration of aerobic exercise.   One measure of how hard you're working is the *minimal intensity threshold.* This is the amount of exertion necessary to increase your heart rate to 60 percent of the maximal predicted heart rate (MPHR) for your age (see Table 3.4). However, older exercisers may reach their minimal intensity threshold at heart rates as low as 45 percent of their MPHR. Figures 3.1 and 3.2 show you how to take your pulse and calculate your heart rate. If your heart rhythm is chronically irregular or you are on medications that slow the heart rate, the best guide to your minimal intensity threshold is not the heart rate itself but the perception of having to breathe harder.

When you exercise above the minimal intensity threshold, the *total* amount of work you do determines how much your aerobic capacity improves. Whether you exercise for a longer period of time at a lower intensity, or for a shorter period with greater effort, the rate of improvement in fitness is comparable as long as you expend the same total amount of energy.

Generally, it's better to exercise longer but at a lower effort level than to do higher-intensity workouts for a shorter period of time. This is because higher-intensity exercise may be uncomfortable, and it's easy to lose interest in an activity that hurts. Furthermore, higher-intensity activity is more likely to cause muscle strains, bursitis, tendinitis, ligament sprains, and even fractures.

Exercising safely.   To improve your aerobic fitness *safely,* the following principles should serve as a guide:

TABLE 3.4   MAXIMAL PREDICTED HEART RATE (MPHR) FOR MEN AND WOMEN

These numbers are only estimates. Maximal predicted heart rate (MPHR) may vary ±15 beats per minute.

AGE	MPHR	AGE	MPHR	AGE	MPHR
22	198	42	178	62	158
24	196	44	176	64	156
26	194	46	174	66	154
28	192	48	172	68	152
30	190	50	170	70	150
32	188	52	168	72	148
34	186	54	166	74	146
36	184	56	164	76	144
38	182	58	162	78	142
40	180	60	160	80	140

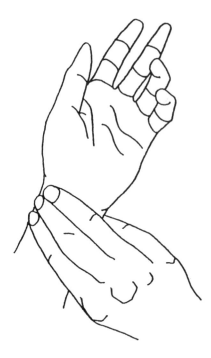

FIGURE 3.1 TAKING YOUR PULSE To feel the radial artery pulse, take the middle three fingers of one hand and press them just below the wrist of your other hand. The fingers should be pressed flat, perpendicular to the outside bone of the forearm.

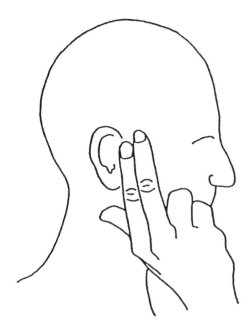

FIGURE 3.2 TAKING YOUR PULSE To feel the temporal artery pulse, press the first two fingers of either hand in the recess in front of the ear on the same side, at the outside end of the cheekbone.

◆ **YOU CAN NEVER START OR ADVANCE YOUR ACTIVITY PROGRAM TOO SLOWLY.**

This is especially important if you are just beginning an activity program or have underlying orthopedic or medical problems. If you have been sedentary, start with five or ten minutes of leisurely walking and then increase the time by two minutes each day until you are walking 20 minutes comfortably. As long as you feel no discomfort at that point, there's little danger in increasing the pace or adding other activities to your exercise program.

◆ **IF IT'S PAINFUL OR UNCOMFORTABLE, REDUCE THE INTENSITY AND DURATION OF YOUR ACTIVITY.**

If there's any question in your mind, stop your exercise program until you consult with a physician. Above all, listen to what your body tells you.

Controlling Weight

Being overweight is a major health problem in the United States. It contributes to the development of coronary artery disease, hypertension, diabetes, high cholesterol, arthritis, gout, and lung disease. In addition, being overweight is an esthetic concern for many people and it can interfere with their emotional well-being.

Most of us aren't aware of how closely we match our daily caloric intake to our energy expenditure. For example, if you take in only an extra 50 calories per day, you will gain five pounds of fat in a year. Fifty calories are found in only a half-can of light beer, two ounces of wine, five saltine crackers, three olives, or four ounces of orange juice.

Optimum health calls for men to have 10 to 20 percent of their weight as body fat and women to maintain 15 to 25 percent body fat. Whether your own weight is a serious health problem can be determined by calculating your body mass index (BMI).

BMI = Weight ÷ (Height)²

Body mass index is calculated in terms of kilograms and meters. First divide your weight in pounds by 2.2. Then divide your height in inches by 39.4 and square that number. Finally, divide the first result by the second result, and that is your BMI.

If you weigh 145 pounds and you are 5 feet 5 inches tall, the calculations go like this:

1. Convert weight in pounds to kilograms: $145 \div 2.2 = 65.9$
2. Convert height in inches to meters: $65 \div 39.4 = 1.65$
3. Square the height in meters: $1.65 \times 1.65 = 2.72$
4. Divide the result in **1** by that in **3**: $65.9 \div 2.72 = 24.2$

The BMI is 24.2.

A BMI between 20 and 35 indicates a "normal" weight and an average risk of death. If your BMI exceeds 30, there is a moderate increase in death rates. With a BMI above 40, the general mortality rate is markedly higher.

If your goal is to lose weight, you need to burn more calories than you take in; aerobic activity should be an integral part of your program. At the same time, take a fresh and honest look at your diet and exercise program. Researchers at the Columbia University Obesity Research Center studied people who were unable to lose weight despite exercising and trying to limit their caloric intake. They found that individuals who were unsuccessful tended to underestimate their caloric intake by an average of 47 percent and overestimated their physical activity by an average of 51 percent.

Focus on the *quantity* of activity, not the intensity of your effort. If you put in the time, you don't have to push yourself to the point of breathlessness or exhaustion. In fact, you use almost the same total amount of energy whether you walk a mile in 24 minutes or in 15 minutes (75 to 80 calories for a 150-pound person); whether you run a mile in 10 minutes or in eight minutes (roughly 120 calories); or whether you bicycle one mile in five minutes or four minutes (about 45 calories). Table 3.5 details the number of calories that people burn during specific aerobic activities.

Building and Strengthening Muscles

There are several good reasons to build muscles and increase your strength. Being stronger means that you can do specific activities more effectively and for a longer period of time before you tire out. Moreover, many people feel that by improving muscle bulk and muscle tone, they enhance their appearance, which makes them feel better about themselves. Whatever your reasons for wanting to increase muscle strength, there are two basic principles that govern a weight training program: *specificity* and *overload*.

First, you develop only the muscles that you *specifically* exercise. If you want to strengthen your legs for skiing, do exercises for your inside (medial), outside (lateral), and front (anterior) thigh muscles. If you wish to improve your forearm and wrist for tennis, work on strengthening those specific muscles in the arm. It's just as important to work the so-called antagonist muscle groups, because at least two opposing muscle groups are involved in all repetitive body movements. (For example, the biceps bend the arms and the triceps straighten them.) Strengthening only one specific muscle group causes an imbalance in muscle strength that can lead to injury. But if your goal is to enhance your overall strength, then you need a well-rounded program of 8 to 10 exercises that involve *all* of the major muscle groups in your body.

Second, to increase your strength, you have to *overload* the muscles. You must push, pull, or lift more than you would in ordinary situations. Any degree of excess load increases your muscular strength. When your exertion approaches your maximum possible effort, you see greater results. Prudence is important, because as you approach the limits of your muscle strength, you also increase the likelihood of tendon, ligament, and muscle injuries.

Intensity and duration of weight training.   According to the American College of Sports Medicine, whether you use resistance machines or free weights, you should perform each specific exercise in a set of 8 to 12 repetitions so that at the end of the set, your strength is nearly exhausted. Increase the amount of weight every one or two weeks as long as you feel comfortable. When you can do at least 12 repetitions of the exercise, you can safely increase the weight.

This moderate program allows you to achieve 70 to 80 percent of the gain that would come with more vigorous and frequent workouts. But remember, as you increase the frequency of your workouts, you also raise the risk of injury.

TABLE 3.5 ESTIMATED CALORIES BURNED PER 20 MINUTES OF ACTIVITY

The number of calories you burn during exercise depends partly on your body weight and partly on the intensity of your effort.

ACTIVITY	WEIGHT 105	WEIGHT 120	WEIGHT 135	WEIGHT 150	WEIGHT 165	WEIGHT 180	WEIGHT 195
Daily activities							
Sleeping	16	20	22	24	26	28	32
Sitting, eating	22	24	28	30	34	36	40
Conversing	26	28	32	36	40	44	46
Office work	36	42	46	52	58	62	68
Aerobic dance							
Low-impact	106	120	136	150	166	180	196
High-impact	154	176	198	220	242	264	286
Alpine skiing							
Moderate	112	128	144	160	176	192	208
Steep	168	192	216	240	264	288	312
Baseball	66	76	84	94	104	112	122
Basketball							
Half-court	84	96	108	120	132	144	156
Full-court	126	144	162	180	198	216	234
Fast-break	210	240	270	300	330	360	390
Bicycling							
8 mph	84	96	108	120	132	144	156
10 mph	98	112	126	140	154	168	182
12 mph	136	154	174	194	212	232	252
15 mph	168	192	216	240	264	288	312
Bowling (while active)	98	112	126	140	154	168	182
Calisthenics							
Light	52	60	66	74	82	88	96
Heavy	140	160	180	200	220	240	260
Cross-country skiing							
3 mph (20 min/mile)	126	144	162	180	198	216	234
4 mph (15 min/mile)	148	168	190	210	232	252	274
5 mph (12 min/mile)	172	198	222	246	272	296	320
6 mph (10 min/mile)	206	234	264	294	322	352	382
8 mph (7.5 min/mile)	238	272	306	340	374	408	442
Fishing							
Bank, boat, ice	42	48	54	60	66	72	78
Standing—waders	64	72	82	90	100	108	118
Walking—waders	92	104	118	130	144	156	170
Football (while active)							
Touch, casual	106	120	136	150	166	180	196
Touch, competitive	168	192	216	240	264	288	312
Golf							
Power cart	42	48	54	60	66	72	78
Pulling cart	66	74	84	94	102	112	122
Carrying clubs	94	106	120	134	146	160	174
Hiking and climbing							
3.5 mph over field	98	112	126	140	154	168	182
3 mph, 40-lb pack	96	108	122	136	150	164	176
Climbing, casual	84	96	108	120	112	144	156
Climbing, vigorous	168	192	216	240	264	288	312

ACTIVITY	WEIGHT 105	WEIGHT 120	WEIGHT 135	WEIGHT 150	WEIGHT 165	WEIGHT 180	WEIGHT 195
Horseback riding							
Sitting to trot	64	72	82	90	100	108	118
Posting to trot	92	104	118	130	144	156	170
Gallop	126	144	162	180	198	216	234
Ice or roller skating							
Recreational	70	80	90	100	110	120	130
Vigorous	140	160	180	200	220	240	260
Jogging and running							
12:00 per-mile pace	140	160	180	200	220	240	260
10:00 per-mile pace	168	192	216	240	264	288	312
9:30 per-mile pace	176	200	226	250	276	300	326
9:00 per-mile pace	184	210	238	264	290	316	342
8:30 per-mile pace	196	224	252	280	308	336	364
8:00 per-mile pace	210	240	270	300	330	360	390
7:30 per-mile pace	218	250	280	312	344	374	406
7:00 per-mile pace	238	272	306	340	374	408	442
6:30 per-mile pace	250	284	320	356	392	428	462
6:00 per-mile pace	274	314	352	392	432	470	510
Martial arts	182	208	234	260	286	312	338
Racquetball and squash							
Social	140	160	180	200	220	240	260
Competitive	210	240	270	300	330	360	390
Rowing and canoeing							
Pleasure/casual	70	80	90	100	110	120	130
Vigorous canoeing	98	112	126	140	154	168	182
Vigorous rowing	210	240	270	300	330	360	390
Sailing	64	72	82	90	100	108	118
Soccer							
Casual	86	96	108	120	132	144	156
Competitive	210	240	270	300	330	360	390
Swimming							
25 yds/min.	84	96	108	120	132	144	156
50 yds/min.	176	200	226	250	276	300	326
Butterfly, 50 yds/min.	196	224	252	280	308	336	364
Tennis							
Singles, social	106	120	136	150	166	180	196
Singles, competitive	154	176	198	220	242	264	286
Doubles, social	80	90	102	114	124	136	148
Doubles, competitive	114	130	148	164	180	196	212
Volleyball							
Recreational	50	56	64	70	78	84	92
Competitive	112	128	144	160	176	192	208
Walking							
24 min/mile pace	42	48	54	60	66	72	78
20 min/mile pace	52	60	66	74	82	88	96
17 min/mile pace	58	68	76	84	92	100	110
5% uphill grade	106	120	136	150	166	180	196
10% uphill grade	140	160	180	200	220	240	260
15% uphill grade	182	208	234	260	286	312	338
15 min/mile pace	79	88	100	110	122	132	144
12 min/mile pace	116	132	150	166	182	200	216
Weight training (circuit)	140	160	180	200	220	240	260

Exercising safely. For building and strengthening muscles, the following guidelines help you proceed safely.

> ◆ **YOU CAN NEVER START OR ADVANCE YOUR WEIGHT-TRAINING PRO-GRAM TOO SLOWLY.**

This is especially important if you've been inactive or have underlying orthopedic or medical problems. Start at a comfortable level with only light weights and advance by five-pound increments every week or two until you are unable to increase the weight.

> ◆ **IF IT'S PAINFUL OR UNCOMFORTABLE, REDUCE THE LOAD—OR STOP THE PARTICULAR EXERCISE ALTOGETHER AND GO TO ANOTHER ONE.**

Your energy and strength, as well as your tolerance for pain and your personal motivation, may vary from day to day. You don't have to match last week's performance with today's. *Listen to your body.*

Reducing Everyday Stress

Exercise is a good way to deal with stress and anxiety. You don't have to exercise at a high intensity to reduce tension. In fact, the best way to achieve a relaxing effect is to do rhythmic noncompetitive "mindless" activity such as walking, jogging, cycling, or swimming at only 30 to 60 percent of your maximal intensity. The important factor here is not thinking about what you're doing, so that you develop a detached state similar to meditation. For some people, doing aerobic activity three times a week reduces hostile, competitive, type-A behavior. However, what is repetitive and relaxing for one person may be boring and tedious for someone else. The bottom line for relieving stress is to find activities that you enjoy.

FOOD AND DRINK FOR EXERCISE

For any activity program, there are two distinct nutritional issues: First, what is the best everyday diet? Second, what should you eat and drink before and during exercise itself? In either case, your diet should

- provide enough energy and fluid for you to exercise efficiently
- satisfy your body's needs for muscle development and tissue repair
- be readily absorbed into your system
- generate waste products that will not impede performance

The best everyday diet is one in which more than 50 percent of total calories comes from carbohydrates, about 10 to 15 percent from protein, and roughly 25 percent from fat (see Table 3.6). You can follow this diet by

- avoiding junk foods and most fatty, fried foods
- eating starches such as rice, potatoes, grains, and pasta
- consuming fresh fruits and vegetables
- eating meat as a side dish rather than as a main course

TABLE 3.6   CALORIES AND SODIUM CONTENT FROM CARBOHYDRATES, PROTEINS, AND FATS IN COMMON FOODS

FOODS	CARBOHYDRATE (cals)	PROTEIN (cals)	FAT (cals)	TOTAL (cals)	SODIUM (mg)
Beverages					
Cola (12-oz. can)	151	0	0	151	14
Diet cola (12-oz. can)	0	0	0	1	60
Whole milk (8 oz.)	44	33	73	150	122
Milk 1% (8 oz.)	45	32	25	102	123
Regular beer (12 oz.)	53	4	0	150	19
Light beer (12 oz.)	20	3	0	100	10
Nonalcoholic beer (12 oz.)	57	3	0	70	9
Orange juice (8 oz., fresh frozen)	104	7	1	112	2
Grapefruit juice (8 oz., fresh)	94	5	3	102	2
Lemonade (8 oz., from frozen)	132	0	1	133	10
Cranberry juice cocktail (8 oz.)	146	0	1	147	10
Distilled spirits, 94 proof (1.5 oz.)	0	0	0	116	0
Wine, red or white (3.5 oz.)	0	0	0	72	0
Grains and Starches					
White rice (1 cup, cooked)	202	16	5	223	2
Potato (baked with skin)	199	19	2	220	16
Pasta and noodles (1 cup, cooked)	148	28	24	200	3
Spaghetti sauce (4 oz., prepared)	77	8	51	136	623
Bagel (1 plain)	124	25	14	163	198
English muffin (1 whole)	104	18	13	135	364
White bread (1 slice)	46	8	10	64	123
Saltines (2 crackers)	36	5	11	26	80
Cornflakes (1 cup)	98	8	2	108	277
Meats and Dairy Products					
Chicken breast (roasted without skin)	0	111	31	142	63
Chicken breast (roasted, with skin)	0	123	70	193	69
Beef (3.5 oz., ground lean)	0	103	172	275	77
Cheese (American/Swiss, 1 oz.)	2/5	25/27	80/75	107	406/440
Yogurt (plain, 8-oz. container)	72	50	38	160	140
Ice cream (vanilla, 1 cup)	129	20	120	269	116
Frozen yogurt (vanilla, 1 cup)	136	26	48	210	130
Snack Foods					
Raisins (⅔ cup)	285	13	4	302	12
Peanuts (2 oz., dry roasted)	48	52	228	328	456
Sunflower nuts (2 oz., dry roasted)	54	44	232	330	436
Potato chips (2 oz.)	120	15	161	296	266
Pretzels (2 oz., salted)	184	22	14	220	902
Corn chips (2 oz.)	134	14	158	306	436
Fast Foods					
Pizza (cheese, 1 slice)	159	63	68	290	698
Quarter-pound cheeseburger	122	126	277	525	1,220
Fried chicken leg (extra crispy)	20	54	99	173	346
Large french fries	174	12	167	353	262
Glazed doughnut	123	8	99	230	200

Caloric Intake

Most recreational exercisers don't burn up enough calories to have the luxury of unlimited food intake. The average adult usually metabolizes between 1,600 and 2,800 calories per day. In contrast, competitive marathoners, triathletes, bicyclists, and endurance swimmers may burn as many as 5,000 calories per day (and must eat constantly to maintain their weight).

Daily Intake of Fluid and Salt

The best way to make sure you have enough fluid in your diet is to drink enough water so that your urine is light in color. But you should minimize caffeinated beverages such as coffee, tea, and colas because they have a diuretic effect. Salt tablets are *not* recommended, and they can be dangerous. Salt depletion is rarely a day-to-day concern as long as you have enough salt in your food to suit your taste. However, if you take diuretic medications or if you have any concerns about salt intake, discuss this with your physician.

Interestingly, your sense of thirst isn't a reliable indicator of your fluid balance and reserve. With exercise, the best way to know if you're taking in enough liquid is to monitor your weight daily. If your weight is down more than one or two pounds after exercising, it's because of fluid loss, and you need to drink more water. This is more important during warm weather, when gradual fluid depletion can affect your energy level as well as your exercise performance.

Food and Drink Before and During Activity

What you should eat and drink prior to activity largely depends on the type of exercise you do. The goal of preexercise nutrition is to build up a reserve of fuel and fluid in a way that will not slow you down. The foods you eat before exercise should be high in carbohydrates, low in fat and protein, low in bulk, and moderate or even low in salt. This is because fatty foods take longer to empty from the stomach and reach the small intestine, where the nutrients are actually absorbed. Moreover, foods that are high in protein and salt can result in water loss through the kidneys, thereby raising the risk of dehydration during subsequent activity.

When you eat is an important part of exercise and weight control. You can control the buildup of body fat more effectively if you consume a significant number of your calories in the morning, in advance of activity. By eating smaller portions distributed throughout the day (rather than isolated large meals), you can improve your cholesterol level and enhance your overall body metabolism. This dietary approach will provide enough fuel for the energy required for most recreational activities.

Nutrition for endurance activities. If you plan a long run or an all-day tennis tournament, don't eat a heavy meal sooner than four hours prior to exercise. A light, high-carbohydrate menu may be consumed two to three hours ahead of activity. Unless you're involved in *continuous* aerobic activity lasting more than three or four hours, proper diet preparation should provide you with sufficient energy reserves. If you're planning a long run or bicycle ride, either for training or a formal race, you can augment your muscle glycogen stores by carbohydrate loading. To learn how to handle carbohydrate loading safely, consult with a sports trainer or coach.

You should also drink at least 16 ounces of water within an hour of vigorous activity. The extra liquid may make you urinate before you exercise, but you can draw on this reserve of fluid during the activity itself. Once you start to exercise, your fluid requirements will depend on the type and duration of exercise and on the heat and humidity that day. For aerobic exercise lasting less than

45 minutes, you usually don't need to drink fluids until you finish. For the following activities, it's vital that you replace the fluid you lose: long-distance running, endurance cycling, prolonged team sports, and consecutive tennis matches. Fluid intake is also crucial when you're exposed to the sun for extensive periods during sailing, golfing, and fishing.

When you try to replace fluids during vigorous activity, you run into problems because you can't stop long enough (if at all) for your body to absorb more than modest amounts of liquid. During vigorous activity, try to take only five to eight ounces of a cold drink at a time and wait at least 10 to 15 minutes between drinks. Cold drinks are recommended because they empty from your stomach more rapidly, and they have the added benefit of cooling you internally.

There are a number of opinions about the specific kind of fluid you should drink immediately before and during exercise. When you sweat, you lose water far out of proportion to salt and potassium. Therefore, the replacement fluid should be dilute. Drinks with high concentrations of salt and sugar will delay the emptying of the stomach and decrease the absorption of the water you need. Sodium concentrations in the blood can even be elevated because of excessive water loss. Salt tablets should be avoided.

Experiment with several different replacement fluids and choose the one that makes you feel the most comfortable and that allows you to exercise the most effectively.

EXERCISING WHEN YOU TRAVEL

Many people like to continue exercising when they travel. Walkers and joggers have the easiest time; hotels in the United States generally offer maps that outline safe walking and jogging routes, and this information is usually available at the front desk or from a concierge. Many large hotels have exercise rooms equipped with weights and aerobic machines, and some have swimming pools. If they don't have these amenities in the building, many hotels arrange for guests to have access to nearby athletic facilities.

You can exercise in your room by doing calisthenics or working with televised exercise programs or tapes. Some hotels even provide exercise equipment such as stationary bikes for you to use in your room. With a modest amount of planning, you should be able to exercise for fitness and relaxation, even when you are traveling.

4

STRETCHING
AND STRENGTHENING

Physical exercise should be a regular part of everyone's life. We all know that with well-conditioned bodies we can participate in daily work and recreational activities with greater ease and comfort. Ligaments and tendons that aren't stretched will inevitably shorten and become stiffer, and muscles that aren't used regularly will soon weaken. By maintaining a regular stretching and strengthening routine, you'll have more fun and be better able to prevent injury.

THE NUTS AND BOLTS OF STRETCHING AND STRENGTHENING

Stretching

The key to effective stretching is slow and sustained force—not rhythmic or jerky movement. Stretch to the point where you feel modest tension in the muscles, then hold the position for a count of 10 to allow the muscles to relax. Increase the effort until you feel further tightness and hold for a count of at least 10. Lasting benefit comes from regular and moderate stretching, not from excessive straining. Get comfortable, breathe slowly, and maintain a relaxed position. Perform any floor exercises on an exercise mat or carpeting.

Strengthening

Whether you do strengthening exercises with or without equipment, the principles are the same: Don't fully straighten your elbows or knees, which "locks" them. Make your motions smooth and continuous to keep tension on the muscles without straining. Maintain steady, slow breathing and don't hold your breath while you're exerting. (If you hold your breath and strain too hard, your blood pressure rises and there's a temporary decrease in blood flowing back to the heart.) Do strengthening exercises in repetitions of eight to 12, although you may want to work up to that number.

DAILY STRETCHING AND STRENGTHENING PROGRAM

The basic program is short and simple, and it requires no equipment. Try to do it every day.

Start the routine by stretching your arms, shoulders, and upper and mid back. Then move to strengthening with push-ups. Do them either against the wall, on the floor with the knees touching the floor, or with legs straight. While you're on the floor, follow with lower-back flexibility and strengthening. Bringing the knee up to the chest, followed by modified sit-ups and pelvic lifts, completes the basic sequence. Figures 4.1 through 4.10 show the daily routine:

> Vertical arm twist stretch (Figure 4.1)
> Neck, shoulder, and arm stretch (Figure 4.2)
> Sideways lean stretch (Figure 4.3)
> Mid- and lower-back and upper chest stretch (Figure 4.4)
> Push-up against the wall (Figure 4.5)
> Bent-knee push-up (Figure 4.6)
> Standard push-up (Figure 4.7)
> Lower-back and buttock stretch (Figure 4.8)
> Bent-knee sit-up (Figure 4.9)
> Pelvic tilt (Figure 4.10)

STRETCHING AND STRENGTHENING FOR FUN AND SAFETY

Those muscles that you use the most are the ones that need the most flexibility. When you increase your flexibility, your muscles are less likely to be pulled or strained during vigorous exercise. Runners must stretch their hamstrings (the muscles in the back of the thigh); throwers require flexibility in their shoulders; and everyone who twists, turns, or maintains a bending-forward posture needs to stretch the muscles of the mid and lower back.

When your goal is having fun and exercising safely, strengthening exercises should focus on the muscles that maintain your posture or your body position during activities. For example, downhill skiers use their thigh and lower-back muscles to stay in a crouch while their knees and legs do the moving. When supporting muscles become fatigued, stability may be lost and movements are less precise and less controlled. There's an increased chance of falling, and for some sports there's a greater likelihood of overuse injuries as well.

The exercises that follow pick up where the daily routine leaves off. They more fully stretch and strengthen your body in four important areas:

> - arms, neck, and shoulders
> - mid and lower back
> - hips and thighs
> - calves and heels

Many people engage in different activities at different times of the year, or they cross-train, alternating their exercises on different days of the week. It is easy to vary a stretching and strengthening program to match activities.

The following exercises are designed with various activities in mind. You can do these routines at home without any special equipment. Do them at least three times a week, according to the nuts-and-bolts guidelines.

ARMS, NECK, AND SHOULDERS

Stretching the Arms, Neck, and Shoulders

Stretching the upper body benefits those who ski (downhill or cross-country), those who swim or do martial arts, and those who play golf, racquet sports, baseball, basketball, or volleyball.

> Vertical arm twist stretch (Figure 4.1)
> Vertical arm stretch (Figure 4.11)
> Neck, shoulder, and arm stretch (Figure 4.2)
> Shoulder shrug (Figure 4.12)
> Outer shoulder (triceps) stretch (Figure 4.13)

Strengthening the Arms, Neck, and Shoulders

Strengthening the arms and upper body benefits those who swim, ski, or bowl, and helps those who play golf, racquet sports, baseball, or basketball.

> Push-up against the wall (Figure 4.5)
> Bent-knee push-up (Figure 4.6)
> Standard push-up (Figure 4.7)
> Wrist curls and reverse wrist curls (Figure 4.14)
> Reverse push-ups (Figure 4.15)

MID AND LOWER BACK

Stretching the Mid and Lower Back

Stretching the mid and lower back benefits those who do aerobic dance, martial arts, or rowing; those who play golf or racquet sports; and those who play baseball, basketball, or volleyball.

> Sideways lean stretch (Figure 4.3)
> Mid and lower back and upper chest stretch (Figure 4.4)
> Complete body stretch (Figure 4.16)
> Mid-back stretch (Figure 4.17)
> Mid-back and neck stretch (Figure 4.18)
> Trunk twist (Figure 4.19)

Strengthening the Mid and Lower Back and Abdomen

Strengthening the back and abdominal muscles provides the most benefit to people who ski, jog, bowl, row, or ride bicycles or horses.

> Bent-knee sit-up (Figure 4.9)
> Pelvic tilt (Figure 4.10)
> Stomach crunches (Figure 4.20)
> Back extensions (Figure 4.21)

HIPS AND THIGHS

Stretching the Hips and Thighs

Stretching the hips and thighs benefits those who jog, cycle, cross-country ski, or do martial arts; and those who play racquet sports, touch football, or soccer.

> Lower-back and buttock stretch (Figure 4.8)
> Groin stretch (Figure 4.22)
> Outer-hip (iliotibial band) stretch (Figure 4.23)
> Front-thigh (quadriceps) stretch (Figure 4.24)
> Back-of-the-thigh (hamstring) stretch (Figure 4.25)

Strengthening the Hips and Thighs

Strengthening the hips and thighs is most important for people who cycle or who ski downhill.

> Lunges (Figure 4.26)
> Minisquats (Figure 4.27)
> Thigh squeezes (Figure 4.28)
> Side leg raises (Figure 4.29)

CALVES AND HEELS

Stretching the Calves and Heels

Stretching the calves and heels benefits those who jog; those who do martial arts or aerobic dance; and those who play racquet sports, touch football, basketball, or volleyball.

> Calf and heel stretch (Figure 4.30)
> Calf and heel stretch (Figure 4.31)

Strengthening the Calves and Ankles

Strengthening the calves and ankles is most important for those who do aerobic dance and those who play basketball or soccer.

> Calf raises (Figure 4.32)
> Ankle push (Figure 4.33)

STRETCHING AND STRENGTHENING FOR SPECIFIC ACTIVITIES

These exercises serve as a nucleus for your stretching and strengthening program, and can prevent the injuries that are most likely to occur. But don't limit your stretching and strengthening to these exercises. Be creative and add those exercises that help you maintain your overall conditioning.

Alpine skiing

Focus on the shoulders, upper arms, the mid and lower back, and the hips (Figures 4.2–4.4, 4.17, 4.18, and 4.24).

Maintaining your body position is the key to keeping under control when skiing downhill. Strengthen the mid and lower back, the hips, and the thighs—particularly the front of the thighs (Figures 4.10, 4.20, 4.21, and 4.26–4.29).

Baseball and Touch Football

Stretch the arms and shoulders, mid and lower back, hip and thigh, and heel and calf (Figures 4.1–4.3, 4.13, 4.19, 4.22–4.25, 4.30, and 4.31).

Basketball and Volleyball

Flexibility in the shoulders, mid and lower back, and legs is essential (Figures 4.1–4.4, 4.8, 4.13, 4.17, 4.23–4.25, 4.30, and 4.31).

Ankle strengthening may help prevent sprains (Figure 4.33).

Cross-Country Skiing

Make sure that the upper arm and shoulder, the mid and lower back, as well as the heel and calves are flexible (Figures 4.1–4.4, 4.8, 4.30, and 4.31).

Lower-back and abdominal strengthening are important for postural support (Figures 4.9, 4.10, 4.20, and 4.21).

Cycling

Work on the lower back, hips, knees, and thighs, and the calves and heels (Figures 4.4, 4.8, 4.23–4.25, 4.30, and 4.31).

For recreational cycling, focus on the mid- and lower-back muscles to provide the proper strengthening support for the posture required for bicycling (Figures 4.17 and 4.21).

Golf

Focus on the upper arms and shoulders as well as the mid and lower back to build greater flexibility (Figures 4.1–4.4, 4.13, 4.18, and 4.19).

Jogging

It's essential to maintain flexibility in the heels and calves, knees, hips, and thighs, and in the mid and lower back (Figures 4.8, 4.17–4.19, 4.23–4.25, 4.30, and 4.31).

Abdominal, mid-back, and lower-back exercises are the most important for building postural strength (Figures 4.9, 4.20, and 4.21).

Racquet Sports

You need to stretch the upper arms and shoulders, mid and lower back, hips and thighs, and heels and calves (Figures 4.2, 4.3, 4.8, 4.13, 4.19, 4.22, 4.25, and 4.31). Strengthening exercises should concentrate on the forearm and ankles for greater support (Figures 4.14 and 4.33).

Rowing

Stretching exercises should focus on the arm and shoulder, mid and lower back, and the hips, legs, and knees (Figures 4.1–4.4, 4.8, 4.13, 4.17, and 4.22–4.24).

For recreational rowers and scullers, the rowing itself is the best strengthening activity.

Swimming

Swimmers must keep the shoulders, hips, and knees flexible (Figures 4.1, 4.2, 4.8, 4.13, and 4.22–4.24).

All swimmers will benefit from strengthening the upper arms (Figures 4.5, 4.6, or 4.7; 4.15).

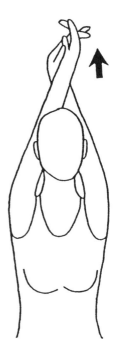

FIGURE 4.1 VERTICAL ARM TWIST STRETCH Twist each arm and clasp your hands gently together. Reach straight up as far as you can without straining. Hold the position for 10 to 15 seconds. You'll feel a stretch on the outside of the arm above and below the elbow.

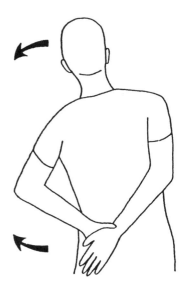

FIGURE 4.2 NECK, SHOULDER, AND ARM STRETCH With your left hand, gently hold your right hand behind your back. Pull the right hand to the left. At the same time, lean your head to the left. Hold for 10 to 15 seconds, then repeat on the opposite side. You'll feel the pulling in the side of the neck, the shoulder, and the back of the arm.

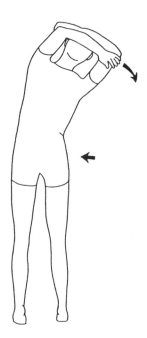

FIGURE **4.3 SIDEWAYS LEAN STRETCH** With your knees slightly bent, gently hold
your arms together behind your head so that your left hand is over the back of the right
elbow. Lean your shoulders sideways to the right. At the same time, push the left hip slightly
out to the side. Hold for 10 to 15 seconds, then repeat on the opposite side. You'll feel the
stretch on the outer side of the body between the shoulder and the top of the hip.

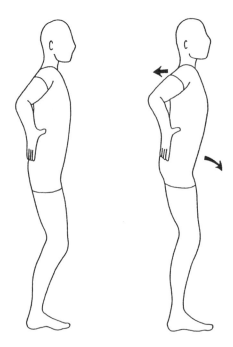

FIGURES **4.4a, 4.4b MID AND LOWER-BACK AND UPPER CHEST STRETCH**
Stand with your knees slightly bent. Place the palms of your hands on the small of your
back, push forward, and rotate your pelvis forward and downward. At the same time, bring
your shoulders back. Hold for at least 10 seconds.

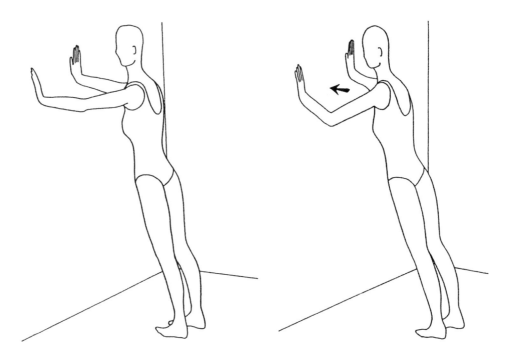

FIGURES 4.5a, 4.5b PUSH-UP AGAINST THE WALL Stand straight with your toes two feet away from the wall and your feet about six inches apart. Slowly lean forward toward the wall, keeping your body straight and bending only your elbows. Push back slowly until your arms are nearly straight. Repeat at least 10 times.

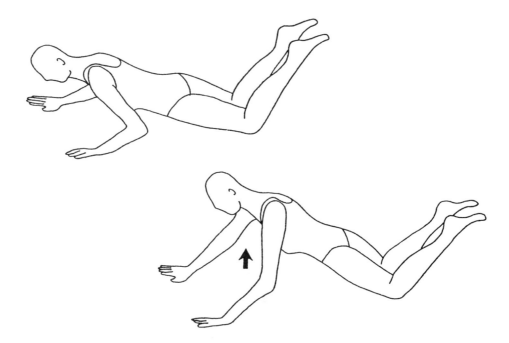

FIGURES 4.6a, 4.6b BENT-KNEE PUSH-UP Lie on the floor with your knees bent. Your hands should be flat on the floor, directly below your shoulders. Keep your fingers pointed straight ahead. Slowly push yourself up by straightening your arms, keeping your body straight. Don't lock your elbows—keep them slightly bent. Look down at the floor to avoid arching your neck. Lower yourself slowly and repeat at least 10 times.

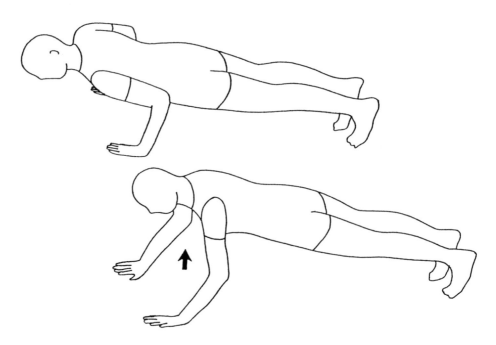

FIGURES 4.7a, 4.7b STANDARD PUSH-UP Start with the palms flat, directly beneath your shoulders. Keep your fingers pointed straight ahead. Slowly raise yourself, keeping your body straight. Don't let your back arch or sag, and don't lock your elbows. Lower yourself slowly and build up to at least 10 repetitions.

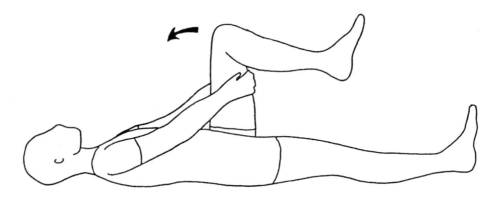

FIGURE 4.8 LOWER-BACK AND BUTTOCK STRETCH Place your hands around the back of your left thigh and bring your knee up as far toward your head as it will go. Hold for at least 15 seconds, and then repeat on the other side. You'll feel the pulling in the upper back of the thigh and in the buttock. Be careful if you have arthritis or cartilage damage in the knee.

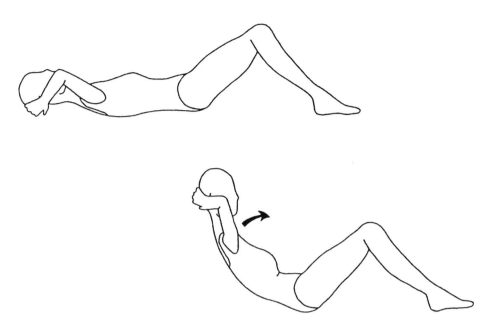

FIGURES 4.9a, 4.9b   BENT-KNEE SIT-UP   To strengthen the upper abdominal muscles, start flat on the floor with your knees bent. Curl upward and forward until your shoulders are off the floor and the ends of your elbows are higher off the floor than the top of your hips. You don't have to bend your neck. Let yourself slowly down. Build up to at least 10 repetitions.

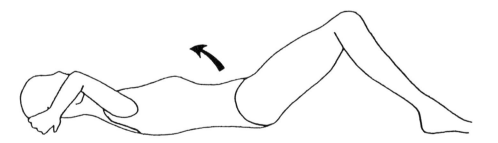

FIGURE 4.10   PELVIC TILT   To strengthen the lower-back and buttocks muscles, squeeze your buttocks together while you lift or rotate your pelvis up and toward your chest. You should feel your lower back press against the floor at the same time. Continue to breathe normally; don't hold your breath. Hold for a count of five and repeat 10 times.

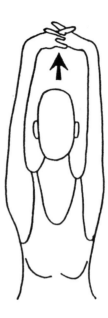

FIGURE 4.11 VERTICAL ARM STRETCH Clasp your hands gently together and reach straight up as far as you can without straining. Hold for 10 to 15 seconds. You'll feel the stretch on the outside of the arms and the top of the shoulders near the neck.

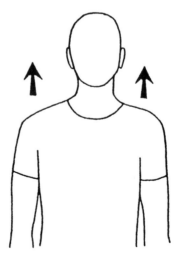

FIGURE 4.12 SHOULDER SHRUG Start with your shoulders and neck relaxed. Then shrug up your shoulders as far as you can and hold for five seconds. Repeat four times.

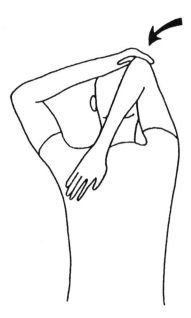

FIGURE 4.13 OUTER-SHOULDER (TRICEPS) STRETCH Reach behind your head and touch the back of your right elbow with your left hand. Use your left hand to push down on the right arm just above the elbow. Hold for 10 to 15 seconds, then repeat with the opposite side. You'll feel the stretch on the upper part of the arm.

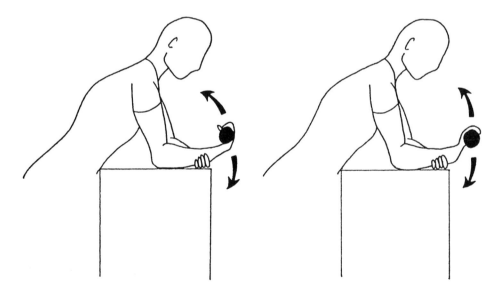

FIGURES 4.14a, 4.14b WRIST CURLS AND REVERSE WRIST CURLS These exercises strengthen the forearm muscles. You can use a one- to three-pound weight or a 16-ounce bottle or can. Rest your right forearm flat on a table (or on your thigh if you're sitting). You can stabilize the forearm by holding it with your left hand. Hold the weight with your right palm facing up. Moving only your wrist, slowly raise and lower the weight 10 times. Do this exercise at least 10 more times with your palm facing down. Repeat the exercise with the left hand.

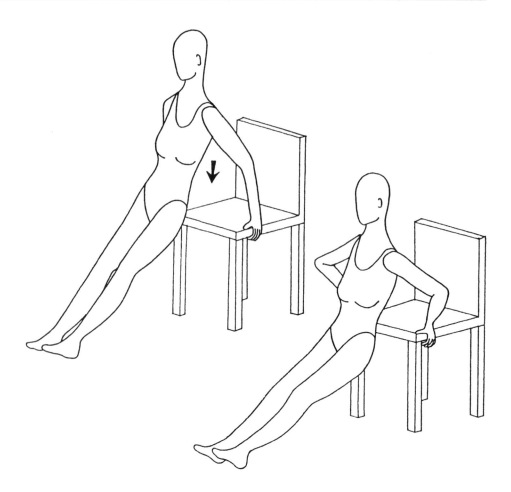

FIGURES 4.15a, 4.15b REVERSE PUSH-UPS These strengthen the arms and upper back. Start as shown in Figure 4.15a. Keep your arms slightly bent so that you don't lock your elbows. Slowly lower your body by bending your elbows. Bend at the waist as well, but keep your legs straight. Slowly lower and raise, and try to work up to at least 10 repetitions. (Your chair should be on carpeting so it doesn't slide.)

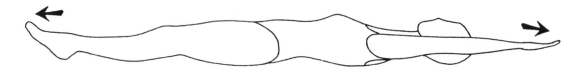

FIGURE 4.16 COMPLETE BODY STRETCH Lying on your back, point your hands and reach as far up beyond the top of your head as you can. At the same time, point your toes downward. Hold for 10 to 15 seconds.

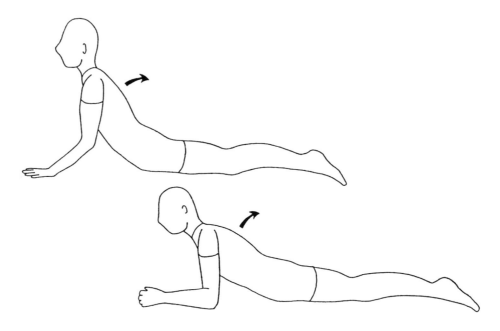

FIGURES 4.17a, 4.17b MID-BACK STRETCH Keep your thighs and pelvis flat on the floor, with your hands below your shoulders. Push up and straighten your arms, then lift up your upper back. Hold for 10 to 15 seconds. If your back is stiff or if you are just beginning, start by resting on your forearms.

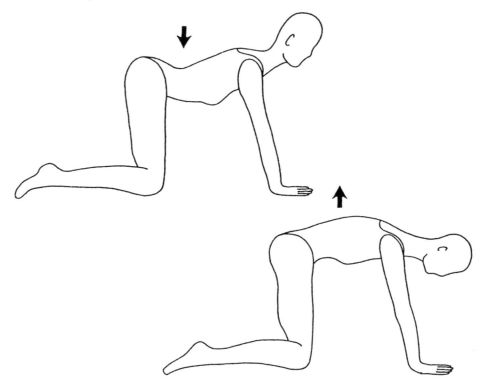

FIGURES 4.18a, 4.18b MID-BACK AND NECK STRETCH   (Omit this stretch if it causes pain in your knees or neck.) On your hands and knees, slowly look up and go into a "sway-back" position. Hold for five seconds. Then slowly look down and raise your mid back. Hold for five seconds. Do four repetitions.

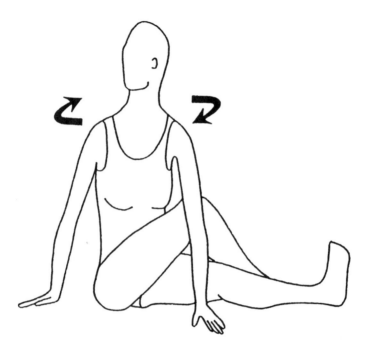

FIGURE 4.19   TRUNK TWIST   Cross your right leg over your left knee and keep the sole of the right foot flat on the floor. Look behind you and twist your torso to the right as far as you can. Hold for 15 seconds, then repeat to the opposite side.

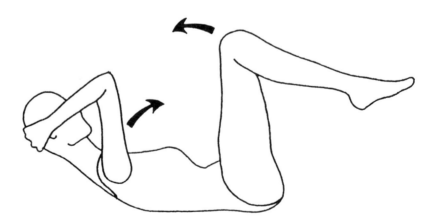

FIGURE 4.20   STOMACH CRUNCHES   To strengthen the lower abdominal muscles, roll your shoulders upward and forward off the floor and raise your knees. Keep your lower back against the floor and use your abdominal muscles to bring your knees up toward your elbows (your knees don't need to touch your elbows). Then release your legs, keeping the knees bent and your feet above the floor. Only your knees and legs move; your shoulders, arms, and back remain still. Start with two repetitions and build up to 10.

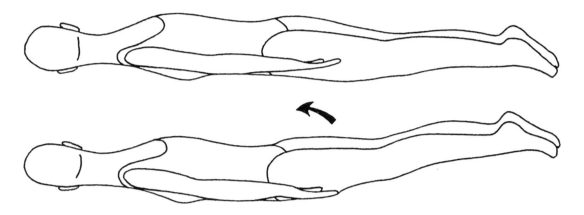

FIGURES 4.21a, 4.21b **BACK EXTENSIONS** (If you have lower-back problems, don't do this exercise without checking with your doctor.) To strengthen the lower-back muscles, squeeze your buttocks together and raise both legs off the floor. Start with two repetitions and work up to 10.

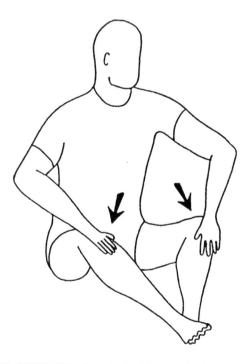

FIGURE 4.22 **GROIN STRETCH** (Don't do this exercise if it causes pain in your hips.) Sit with the soles of your feet touching. Push down on your knees and hold for 10 to 15 seconds. You'll feel the stretch in the inside of the thighs.

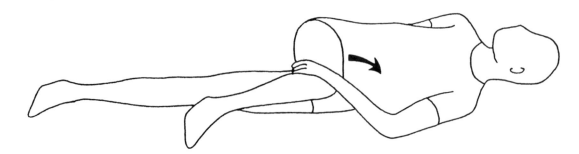

FIGURE 4.23 OUTER-HIP (ILIOTIBIAL BAND) STRETCH Lie on your back and bring your right knee across the left leg. With your left hand on the back of your right thigh, pull up and out to the left. Hold for 15 seconds. Repeat with the other leg. You'll feel the stretch on the outside of the hip.

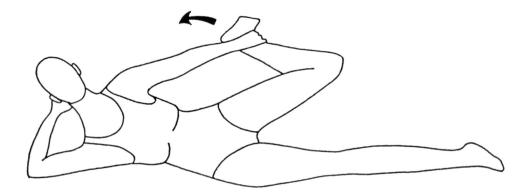

FIGURE 4.24 FRONT-THIGH (QUADRICEPS) STRETCH Lie on your right side and with your left hand on the top of your left foot. Pull back. Hold for 15 seconds, then repeat on the other side. You'll feel the stretch in the front of the thigh.

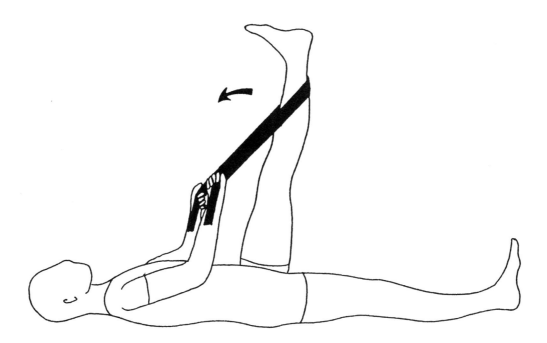

FIGURE 4.25 BACK-OF-THE-THIGH (HAMSTRING) STRETCH Lie on your back. Loop a belt or an old tie around the back of your left calf and pull back toward your head until you feel tightness in the back of your thigh. Count to 10, then pull more firmly to stretch the back of the thigh. Hold for 15 seconds, then repeat with the other leg.

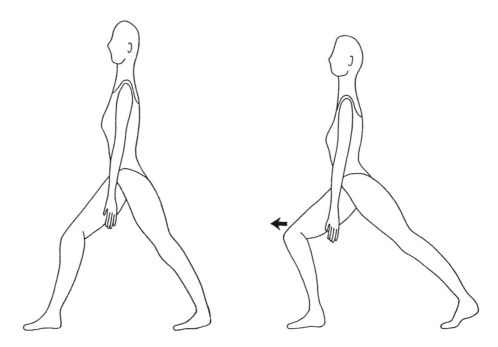

FIGURES 4.26a, 4.26b LUNGES To strengthen the muscles in the front of the thigh (quadriceps), start with your right foot about two feet in front of your left foot. With your left leg straight, slowly bend your right knee. Your left heel will naturally lift from the floor. Return to the starting position and repeat at least 10 times. Do it with the other side.

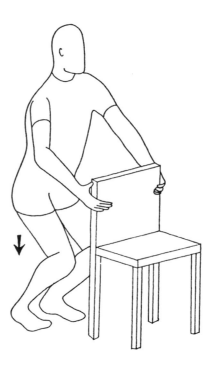

FIGURE 4.27 MINISQUATS To strengthen the front of the thighs, hold on to the back of a chair and slowly lower yourself. Keep your back straight as you bend your legs. Your heels may lift off the floor. Repeat at least 10 times.

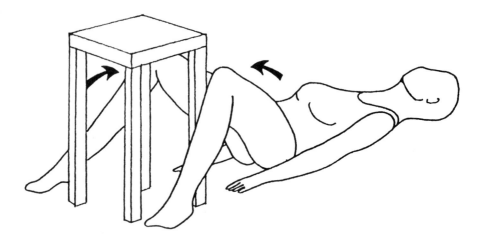

FIGURE 4.28 THIGH SQUEEZES This exercise strengthens the inner muscles of the thighs. Lie flat on the floor with your knees bent and a stool or chair between your upper calves. Squeeze your thighs together and hold for five seconds. Repeat at least five times.

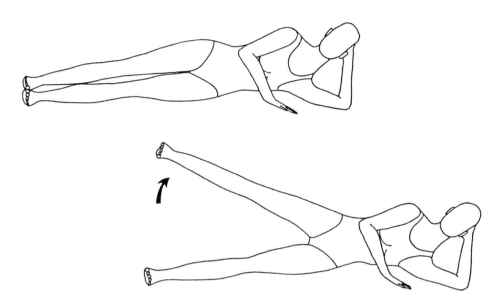

FIGURES 4.29a, 4.29b SIDE LEG RAISES Lie on your left side with your right leg straight. Slowly raise the right leg, keeping it straight. Lower it gradually and repeat at least 10 times to strengthen the outer hip muscles. Be sure that your hips are stacked one on top of the other; don't lean forward or back. Repeat on the other side.

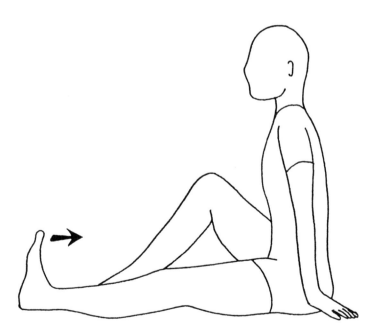

FIGURE 4.30 CALF AND HEEL STRETCH Sit with your right leg bent and your left leg straight. Flex your left foot as hard as you can and hold for 15 seconds. Repeat on the other side.

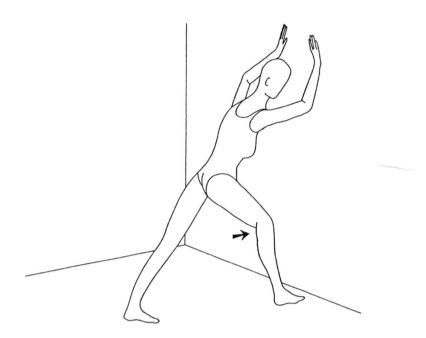

FIGURE 4.31 CALF AND HEEL STRETCH   Stand with your right foot flat on the floor six to eight inches from the wall. Keep your left foot flat on the floor with your leg extended behind you. Point your toes straight ahead. Keeping your feet flat on the floor at all times, and keeping the left leg straight, bend your right knee closer to the wall. Hold for 15 seconds. Repeat with the opposite leg.

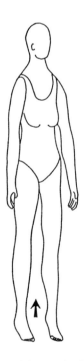

FIGURE 4.32 CALF RAISES   Stand with your back straight and your knees slightly bent for balance. (You may hold on to a chair.) Slowly stand on tiptoes, then let yourself down. Keep a slow easy movement and repeat at least 10 times.

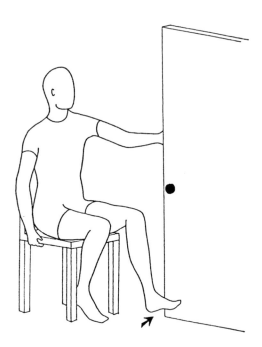

FIGURE 4.33 ANKLE PUSH Sit in a chair in front of an open door. Place the outside of your left foot against the door. Hold the door with your left hand and push against the door with your foot for at least 10 seconds. Repeat with the door against the *inside* of the left foot. Do the same exercises with both sides of the right foot.

5

EXERCISING SAFELY
WITH MEDICAL CONDITIONS

Any medical condition can affect your ability to be active, and you may need to tailor your activity program to fit your special medical needs. Nevertheless, there are safe recreational activities you can and should do to fulfill the exercise guidelines of the American College of Sports Medicine (see chapter 3). In fact, for hypertension, coronary artery disease, osteoporosis, and many orthopedic problems, exercise is an important part of treatment.

Whether a health problem is acute (cold, urinary tract infection), or chronic (heart disease, diabetes), there are specific questions you should consider.

- Which activities might aggravate the problem?
- What are the early warning signs that complications may be developing?
- Which activities may actually improve the condition?

If you have an ongoing medical condition, your quality of life will be enhanced by a prudent flexibility, strengthening, and aerobic exercise program.

BONE AND JOINT DISORDERS

Bone and joint diseases affect over 45 million Americans, most of whom are past the age of 40. Approximately 5 million people in this country have rheumatoid arthritis and roughly 40 million have osteoarthritis.

The word *arthritis* literally means "inflammation of the joint," and this is literally true of rheumatoid arthritis. With *rheumatoid arthritis,* the inner lining of the joint (synovial tissue) is inflamed. This causes heat, redness, swelling, and sometimes the destruction of joints. Rheumatoid arthritis is a disease of the entire body. It can cause fever, weight loss, malaise, and weakness, and powerful anti-inflammatory drugs are often needed to control it. The hands (mainly the knuckles, not the finger joints), the feet, and the knees—as well as other joints—may be involved, usually to the same degree on both sides of the body.

Osteoarthritis isn't so much an inflammation of the joints as a deterioration of the shock-absorbing cartilage that covers the ends of the bones. The skin overlying the joint may be warm, and the joint is usually swollen. But usually there's stiffness and pain, especially when the joint is used or bears weight. As the cartilage breaks down, bony outgrowths (bone spurs) form along the outside of the joint. Bits of cartilage can even break off inside the knee to produce a grinding sensation or a locking of the joint with movement. Osteoarthritis is found in joints that are heavily used—for example, the middle and ends of the fingers, the base of the thumb, the hips, the knees, and throughout the spine. Yet badly deformed osteoarthritic joints may be entirely free of pain.

General Precautions

When signs of inflammation are present (swelling, heat, pain), curtail active exercise of the involved joints. Give your joints sufficient time to rest and recover after exercise. Apply ice packs to localized areas of inflammation and/or take anti-inflammatory medication to allow more comfortable movement. After the signs of inflammation subside, resume those activities that allow joint movement without subjecting the joints to excessive impact and strain. However, if any new aching, swelling, or stiffness persists after 24 hours of rest, there may be additional joint irritation and damage, and you should consult a physician.

Recommended Exercises

Exercise is an essential part of an arthritis therapy program. A stretching, strengthening, and overall fitness regimen helps maintain joint and cartilage function, strengthens bones and ligaments, prevents joint deformities, and enhances your quality of life.

If you have arthritis, stretching and strengthening exercises are easier if you do them on a chair or in a swimming pool.

Chair exercises. Use any basic chair you have at home. The key to achieving the best results is to exercise for a short period of time. Exercises may be mildly uncomfortable but should not be continued if they cause severe pain (Figures 5.1–5.7).

Water exercises. Stretching and strengthening exercises done in the water are effective for people with arthritis (Figures 5.8–5.13).

Arthritis of the Knee

The arthritic knee is vulnerable to the stress of any exercise. High-impact activities may bring on chemical crystal formation in the knee joint, causing a painful inflammation and swelling (pseudogout).

Exercise precautions. The knee is exposed to heavy loads and to pressures with jogging or racquet sports. It is also susceptible to strains with vigorous cycling. When pain, swelling, or stiffness occurs, reduce the intensity, duration, and frequency of exercise—or stop the activity altogether. Anti-inflammatory drugs may be helpful, and corticosteroids (cortisone) can be injected directly into the joint when pain and swelling are severe. If you receive a corticosteroid injection, be sure to ask your doctor how soon you may safely resume exercise activities.

Recommended activities.   Swimming provides excellent aerobic exercise for arthritis of the knee. Running in the deep end of a swimming pool (wear a buoyancy vest) and cross-country skiing are good aerobic alternatives.

Arthritis of the Hip

Degeneration of the hip joint (osteoarthritis) is more prevalent with increasing age. Pain may be felt in the hip, groin, or knee.

Exercise precautions.   Jogging and racquet sports often bring on pain and stiffness in the arthritic hip. Avoid activities such as martial arts or racquetball, which require quick movements. Refrain from jumping sports such as basketball and volleyball.

Recommended activities.   Swimming (except for the breaststroke), walking, and cross-country skiing are the best tolerated aerobic exercises.

Arthritis of the Spine

Degenerative arthritis of the spine is more prevalent in people over 60. Stiffness or aching in the back during and after exercise is common.

Exercise precautions.   Direct strains from weight training, aerobic impact activities, and repeated twisting and bending can worsen symptoms. Occasionally, bone spurs press against nerves in the lower back, a condition called spinal stenosis. This can bring on pain during activities when you stand up straight or bend backward.
   Degenerative changes in the neck (cervical spine) may cause a grinding sensation and discomfort when you turn your head. Bone spurs on the cervical vertebrae may put pressure on adjacent nerves, causing shooting pains or aching in the shoulders, arms, and hands. If pains in the neck, arms, lower back, or legs are aggravated by activity, check with your doctor before you proceed with an exercise program.

Recommended activities.   Walking, jogging, cycling, swimming, and racquet sports are okay as long as you can do them comfortably. If a stiff neck makes it hard to lift your head out of the water to breathe when swimming, use a mask and snorkel.

Arthritis of the Shoulder, Arm, and Hand

You use your shoulders, arms, and hands for so many activities that when arthritic symptoms develop, they affect not only your exercise activities but your daily routines as well.

Exercise precautions.   Rowing, racquet sports (including tennis, squash, and racquetball), swimming strokes such as the butterfly and crawl, and throwing activities are all ill-advised. If you have arthritis in the wrists and hands, bowling, skiing, rowing, and especially weight training may worsen your symptoms. The thumb is a particularly vulnerable joint, and pain and swelling may also be aggravated by sailing and fishing, depending on the amount of stress.

Recommended activities. Jogging is permissible as long as your feet, knees, and hips are not arthritic as well. Make basic flexibility and strengthening exercises a part of your program (see chapter 4).

To maintain flexibility in your hands and wrists, do the following exercises twice a day, if possible.

Stretching the Fingers

Place your hands palms-down on a flat surface and hold your fingers tightly together. Then spread your fingers out as far as you can. Hold for five seconds. Slide your fingers back together again. Repeat the pattern five times.

Stretching the Wrists

Interlock your fingers with your palms touching, and bend your elbows. Hold your clasped hands in front of you as if praying. Push the left hand, and bend the wrist back with your right hand. Hold for five seconds, then repeat the other way. Do the sequence five times.

Fingertip Touch

Hold your left hand up in front of you with your elbow bent. Gently move the tip of your thumb to touch the tip of each finger, making the round shape of the letter O. Try to straighten the fingers not making the O. If needed, use the right hand to help. Repeat the exercise with the right hand.

Artificial Knees and Hips

Each year American physicians replace 100,000 arthritic knees and 160,000 arthritic hips. Typically, artificial joints last for 10 years or so before they begin to loosen and cause problems with pain and instability. Excessive wear and tear from activity shortens the life span of prosthetic knees and hips. This can pose a problem, because second operations tend to be more difficult and less successful than initial joint replacements.

Exercise precautions. Make sure your activity program is approved by your orthopedic surgeon.

Recommended activities. After full recovery and rehabilitation from a knee or hip replacement, consider activities such as walking on level ground, recreational cycling, cross-country skiing, swimming, and rowing. Follow the guidelines recommended by the American College of Sports Medicine (see chapter 3).

Osteoporosis

Osteoporosis is a loss of bone-mineral content (literally, a diffuse thinning of bone). It affects men in their eighties as well as many younger, postmenopausal women.

Exercise precautions.   Although osteoporosis per se doesn't affect exercise capability, it definitely increases the likelihood of fractures. Avoid activities that require jumping or those that may cause serious falls.

Recommended activities.   Exercise is an essential component of the treatment for osteoporosis. A combination of upper- and lower-body exercises will help increase bone density. Walking and running strengthen the bones of the feet, legs, pelvis, and lower spine. Push-ups, isometric exercises, and weight training benefit the shoulders and arms. Combine proper exercising for osteoporosis, and follow the guidelines of the American College of Sports Medicine (see chapter 3) to attain maximum benefit.

Exercise for Osteoporosis

Lower body (legs, pelvis, and spine).   It's essential to do exercises for the lower body that involve activities in which your legs support your body weight. To build lower-body strength, choose among the following activities: walking, hiking, jogging, any running sport (basketball or soccer), aerobic dance, or any racquet sport.

Upper body (upper chest, shoulders, and arms).   You can do any of the following exercises at home.
   Pushing exercises. Start with either the push-up against the wall (Figure 4.5), bent-knee push-up (Figure 4.6), or the standard push-up (Figure 4.7). For the arms and upper back, do reverse push-ups (Figure 4.15). Continue with arm pushes (Figure 8.7).
   Movement exercises. To strengthen the forearm and wrist, do wrist curls and reverse wrist curls (Figure 4.14).

Resistance and weight training.   If you exercise at a fitness center or a gym, working out with resistance machines and weight training will increase bone density. Initially, do any weight training exercises under supervision.

BLOOD DISORDERS

Anemia

A low red blood cell count (anemia) reduces the oxygen-carrying capacity of the blood.

Exercise precautions.   If you experience increased fatigue, consult your doctor. Anemia may also worsen the symptoms of coronary artery disease. When the anemia is due to sickle-cell trait or sickle-cell disease, avoid vigorous exertion at high altitudes because blood clots can form in the spleen. The pain may be disabling and require immediate medical care.

Recommended activities.   Anemia itself shouldn't prevent you from being physically active. However, the reduced oxygen-carrying capacity of the blood decreases stamina and can cause fatigue. Stay active as long as you feel comfortable.

Blood-Clotting Problems

Two conditions hamper blood coagulation: (1) a low concentration of blood-clotting cells (platelets), or deficiencies in one or more of the blood-clotting proteins; or (2) use of medications (warfarin, aspirin, or heparin) that inhibit blood from clotting.

Exercise precautions. Avoid contact sports such as football and martial arts. Take extra care with skiing or cycling, because there's a significant risk of falls and traumatic injury.

Recommended activities. Try low-impact activities such as walking, rowing, and swimming. If you jog, go at an easy pace and run on soft surfaces to keep impact and bruising to a minimum.

STOMACH AND INTESTINAL DISORDERS

The gastrointestinal tract includes the esophagus, stomach, small intestine, and colon (large intestine). Exercise affects how your stomach empties and the rate at which nutrients are absorbed from the intestinal tract. It can also affect the colon by stimulating bowel activity.

Heartburn and Hiatal Hernia

Heartburn is the sensation that occurs when stomach acid washes back (refluxes) into the esophagus. *Hiatal hernia,* a bulging of the stomach up through the diaphragm into the chest, is a common cause of acid reflux and heartburn.

Exercise precautions. Heartburn tends to come and go. It may occur one day and not the next, even with the same amount of exercise. Avoid eating prior to activity, especially fatty foods that tend to delay the emptying of the stomach. Aspirin or ibuprofen taken for aches and pains can irritate an already inflamed stomach lining, increasing the risk of bleeding. Use caution with antacids. They can have a laxative effect, and along with dehydration, they can lead to the formation of kidney stones. Medications that decrease acid production such as cimetidine (*Tagamet*) and ranitidine (*Zantac*) can be very helpful for preventing exercise-related stomach symptoms. Check with your physician.

Recommended activities. Any activity is permissible. When heartburn or acid distress occurs, cut down on the intensity of your activity until you feel better.

Peptic Ulcer

A peptic ulcer is a sore in the lining of the stomach or the duodenum.

Exercise precautions. Exhausting aerobic exercise may aggravate peptic ulcers. Moreover, if you take aspirin or ibuprofen for aches and pains, the ulcer is more likely to bleed.

Recommended activities. Any activity that doesn't make you feel worse is fine.

Acute and Chronic Hepatitis

Liver inflammation (hepatitis) may be caused by viral infections or by irritation from drugs and chemicals.

Exercise precautions.   Liver disease can affect your stamina and endurance. Avoid dehydration, and don't exercise to exhaustion. Consult your doctor if you have any questions.

Recommended activities.   As long as you feel okay, there are no limitations on your activities.

Gallstones

Bile can coalesce to form stones in the gallbladder. Gallstones may block the bile ducts, or they may lead to inflammation of the gallbladder.

Exercise precautions.   See your doctor if you feel persistent pain in the right or middle part of the upper abdomen. You may also feel pain straight through to your back and in your right shoulder.

Recommended activities.   Gallstones shouldn't affect your ability to be active, unless you experience pain during exercise.

Crohn's Disease and Ulcerative Colitis

Crohn's disease and ulcerative colitis are chronic inflammations of the large and small intestine (inflammatory bowel diseases).

Exercise precautions.   See your doctor if you notice any change or worsening of cramps, diarrhea, or rectal bleeding. Avoid dehydration by drinking plenty of water before and after activity.

Recommended activities.   You can engage in any activity as long as you feel comfortable.

Spastic Colon

Intermittent intestinal cramping and bloating that come on for no apparent reason are symptoms of spastic colon.

Exercise precautions.   Aerobic exercises can bring on abdominal cramping and diarrhea. Up to 40 percent of runners feel the urge to have a bowel movement at some point during their run. These sensations are more pronounced with spastic colon. Usually, good fluid intake and sufficient fiber in the diet help prevent symptoms. However, for some people, eating too much fiber may actually aggravate the symptoms of spastic colon during exercise. If this is the case, cut down on cereals and pulpy fruits when you're active. If milk and ice cream bring on bloating, flatulence, or diarrhea with exercise, try either lactose-reduced milk or supplemental lactase enzymes, or remove milk and ice cream from your diet. Unsupervised use of antispasmodic medications to slow intestinal cramping isn't advised. If symptoms persist despite changes in your exercise program or diet, discuss this with your doctor.

Recommended activities. There are no restrictions on physical activity. If early-morning activity causes problems, exercise later in the day.

Hernias and Hemorrhoids

Hernias are bulges that develop in the abdominal wall, around the navel, in the groin, or at the site of previous abdominal surgery. They develop because of weakness and strain in the connecting tissues. *Hemorrhoids* are swollen rectal veins.

Exercise precautions. Be cautious with weight training, sit-ups, leg lifts, and similar exercises, because any straining may cause the weakened tissues to stretch even more. Breathe evenly and avoid straining. Be cautious with bicycle or horseback riding if hemorrhoids are severe. If you feel any discomfort during exercise, consult with a surgeon or your physician.

Recommended activities. Aerobic activities shouldn't seriously aggravate a hernia or hemorrhoids. Follow the American College of Sports Medicine guidelines (see chapter 3).

HEART AND BLOOD VESSEL DISORDERS

There are few health issues that generate more concern for adults who exercise than the risks of heart and blood vessel disorders. People who have high blood pressure, coronary artery disease, irregular heartbeat, and other heart and circulation problems want to live normal lives, and part of a normal life is being physically active.

High Blood Pressure (Hypertension)

One in four Americans—an estimated 58 million people—has high blood pressure.

Exercise precautions. Avoid straining during weight training, because "pumping iron" can temporarily raise blood pressure to alarming levels. Be aware of any precautions imposed by the medications you're taking (see chapter 6).

Recommended activities. Aerobic activities such as walking, jogging, cycling, rowing, dancing, or swimming actually help reduce your blood pressure. Try to sustain aerobic exercise for at least 15 to 20 minutes three times a week.

Coronary Artery Disease

Cholesterol deposits in the coronary arteries (coronary artery disease) can block the flow of blood to the heart muscle, and they are the major cause of heart attacks. Heart muscle that is deprived of blood and oxygen for less than a minute or two usually suffers no permanent damage. But if the blockage lasts for more than a few minutes, the result is a heart attack.

Exercise precautions.   If you have the following symptoms when you exercise, see your doctor.

- chest pain or pressure
- aching in the jaw or neck, pain across the shoulders and back, or pain down the left arm or both arms
- any other sensation that typically comes on with exertion and is relieved promptly by rest

Many people who have coronary artery disease do not have typical symptoms. If you have multiple risk factors for coronary artery disease (see chapter 1) and if you have any of the following symptoms, you should be evaluated by a physician before starting or continuing an activity program.

- dizziness or light-headedness
- any abnormality of the heart rhythm
- the recurrence of any particular sensation that in the past has been associated with heart problems

Recommended activities.   If you've had a heart attack, bypass surgery, dilation of a coronary artery blockage (angioplasty), or a positive stress test, it's vital that you start and advance your activity program under medical supervision. Muscle strengthening and regular aerobic activity such as walking, cycling, rowing, jogging, and swimming are important components of an effective treatment and prevention program. Ask your doctor whether you need to be in a medically supervised exercise class (cardiac rehabilitation program).

Congestive Heart Failure

A history of hypertension, heart attacks, coronary artery disease, heart-valve abnormalities, and viral infections, as well as the long-term toxic effects of alcohol, can all weaken the heart. Some people with congestive heart failure have fluid accumulation in the legs and feet (edema) or shortness of breath at rest or with minimal movement.

Exercise precautions.   Avoid the added environmental stress of heat, cold, or humidity. Be alert to any of the following symptoms: dizziness, light-headedness, palpitations, chest pain, or continued shortness of breath after you stop exercise. See your doctor, because you may need an adjustment of your medications or activity program.

Recommended activities.   A low-level aerobic activity program such as "mall walking" or riding a stationary bike may improve fitness and stamina.

Premature Heartbeats

It's common to have an occasional "thumping" in the chest, even if your heart is normal. You may not even be aware that your heartbeat is irregular until a doctor informs you, or you notice it when you check your pulse. Exercise stress testing or prolonged monitoring of the heart rhythm (Holter monitoring) helps to determine whether abnormal heart rhythms pose a threat.

Exercise precautions. See your doctor if you have any light-headedness or dizziness during exercise. If you have coronary artery disease, assume that the combination of exercise and irregular heart rhythms is dangerous until further evaluation shows that exercise is safe.

Recommended activities. In the absence of underlying coronary artery disease, premature beats of the heart are usually harmless and often disappear during exercise. Any activity is permissible. Follow the guidlelines of the American College of Sports Medicine (see chapter 3).

Atrial Fibrillation

Atrial fibrillation is a very irregular heart rhythm that results in at least a 15 percent loss in heart pumping efficiency. This abnormal heart rhythm can occur in people who don't have any coronary artery or heart muscle disease.

Exercise precautions. Warfarin (*Coumadin*) is often prescribed to prevent clots from forming in the nonpumping upper heart chambers. If you take warfarin, avoid contact sports such as football and basketball, and take extra care with alpine skiing, cycling, and horseback riding, where falls may cause injury and bleeding. Check with your doctor if you feel light-headed, experience chest discomfort, or notice a change in your exercise capability.

Recommended activities. In the absence of any other heart abnormality or underlying medical condition, you may exercise without restriction. Nevertheless, atrial fibrillation may diminish your aerobic stamina. Walking, golf, swimming, and other noncontact activities are generally both safe and beneficial.

Pacemakers

Heart pacemakers are implanted to prevent seriously low heart rates. The pacemaker battery is usually implanted below the collarbone in the upper chest or under the skin in the upper abdomen. Wires extend under the skin and through the veins to make contact with the heart muscle.

Exercise precautions. Weight lifting or other activities that may directly irritate the site of the pacemaker battery should be performed cautiously or avoided. If you experience light-headedness or palpitations during exercise, consult with your physician for further evaluation.

Recommended activities. You can participate in any kind of activity as long as you have the approval of your physician.

Heart Murmurs

A heart murmur may or may not represent a problem with a heart valve.

Exercise precautions. If you experience a thumping in your chest (palpitations), chest discomfort, shortness of breath, or any change in your exercise capability, check with your physician before you proceed.

Recommended activities. If you've been told you have a heart murmur, ask your physician whether there are any limitations on your exercise program.

Hardening of the Arteries and Poor Circulation

Cholesterol plaques (atherosclerosis) in the blood vessels of the abdomen and legs may obstruct blood flow to such an extent that walking becomes painful. Cramping often occurs in the calf or occasionally in the thigh; it comes on with walking or jogging and goes away when you stand and rest. Most often the pain involves only one leg—and it's the same leg each time.

Exercise precautions. Avoid hot soaks in a bath or whirlpool, which can damage the tissues of the feet. Consult with your physician when pain comes on with less exertion, persists after stopping, or occurs at rest, or if you experience unexplained sores on the feet or toes.

Recommended activities. Walk until discomfort occurs and rest until it stops, then start again. This way you help to build up alternative circulatory pathways in the legs. Well-fitted and well-cushioned walking shoes are crucial to prevent damage to the skin from impact and rubbing. Augment the program with pool exercises or sitting flexibility exercises. When walking or jogging is difficult, you may still enhance overall aerobic fitness by swimming and cycling.

Varicose Veins

Prominent veins on the surface of the legs, or varicose veins, may be caused by years of standing at work, previous pregnancies, prior vein inflammation (phlebitis), vein scarring following a fracture or other leg injury, or previous vein removal (with coronary bypass surgery). Discomfort is usually felt after a long period of standing or sitting. Symptoms often improve when the legs are elevated.

Exercise precautions. Typically, varicose veins are more of a discomfort and an annoyance than a serious threat to your health. Avoid wearing compression shorts or tight abdominal binders that inhibit drainage of blood from the legs and may cause swelling and discomfort. See your doctor if skin sores develop on the legs and fail to heal; if there's tenderness, pain, or redness over a vein; or if there's persistent swelling in the feet and ankles. Avoid jogging, stair or step exercises, and high-impact aerobics.

Recommended activities. Swimming is the most desirable form of aerobic activity, followed closely by biking and rowing. Most people with varicose veins are able to walk comfortably. Elastic stockings may provide further support and comfort.

KIDNEY AND BLADDER DISORDERS

Kidney Stones

Kidney stones develop when concentrations of minerals such as calcium become so great that they combine to form stones in the urine. The pain is severe, usually starting in one side of the back or abdomen and traveling to the groin on the same side.

Exercise precautions.   Avoid high-protein diets, excessive calcium intake, and the frequent use of antacids—all of which increase the risk of stone formation. Drink plenty of water before and after exercise, especially in hot and humid weather. Try to drink enough water to keep the urine dilute (light in color), which will reduce the likelihood of stone formation.

Recommended activities.   There are no restrictions on exercise. If symptoms arise, stop exercise and contact your doctor.

Bladder Infection (Cystitis)

Cystitis is inflammation of the bladder, usually the result of an infection.

Exercise precautions.   Avoid vigorous exercise if you feel sick or feverish. If you're taking an antibiotic to treat the cystitis, check to see if it imposes any limitations on activity (see chapter 6). If frequent or urgent urination, pain, or burning persists or worsens, see a physician. Drink plenty of water or diluted cranberry juice to "wash out" the bladder.

Recommended activities.   Activity per se shouldn't affect the course of uncomplicated cystitis.

Prostate Enlargement

Men who have prostate enlargement often need to urinate more frequently. There may be a sense of urgency that allows for little time to reach a lavatory.

Exercise precautions.   If you have a prostate infection (prostatitis), avoid cycling and horseback riding, which may cause irritation from the impact of the seat or saddle. With prostate enlargement, the urgent and more frequent urination creates logistical concerns.

Recommended activities.   The presence of an enlarged prostate shouldn't otherwise affect your exercise plans.

Urinary Incontinence

Involuntary loss of urine (incontinence) affects women more often than men and becomes more prevalent as people get older.

Exercise precautions.   Slightly more than one-third of women who either jog or engage in high-impact aerobics experience some incontinence during exercise. While exercise per se doesn't cause weakened bladder support, urinary leakage is often aggravated by running and jumping.

Recommended activities.   Concentrate on low-impact activities such as bicycling or swimming. Try water strength and stretching exercises (Figures 5.8–5.13).

DIABETES AND OBESITY

Diabetes (Diabetes Mellitus)

Roughly 14 million people in the United States have diabetes. These individuals either don't produce enough insulin or the insulin that they do make doesn't work effectively. Nerve damage and circulatory problems often accompany diabetes. Diabetics are more likely to develop kidney damage, insufficient blood flow to the legs, and blockage in the coronary arteries, and also are prone to nerve degeneration in the legs and feet.

Exercise precautions.   Well-fitting athletic shoes and good foot care are essential. Extremes of heat and cold may also aggravate blood vessel and nerve damage. Take extra care under these conditions. The greatest concern is low blood sugar (hypoglycemia) during or after activity. Dizziness, cold sweats, apprehension, and loss of consciousness can indicate low blood sugar. Medications such as beta blockers (see chapter 6), however, can mask some of the symptoms. Moreover, some people may experience only confusion and weakness. Follow these practical measures.

- Test your blood sugar before and after exercise. Don't exercise until the blood sugar falls below 250 milligrams per deciliter (mg/dl). If blood sugar is in the normal-to-low range of 70 to 125 mg/dl, consume readily absorbed carbohydrates before exercising and have them available during activity as well.
- In order to coordinate exercise, diet, and insulin injections, try to exercise at roughly the same time each day. An ideal time is in the morning after a small snack and before your morning insulin injection. Avoid exercising in the evening, because of the risk of delayed falls in blood sugar during sleep.
- Be prepared to adjust the insulin dose as time goes on. Coordinate this with your physician.
- Inject insulin into the abdomen, as opposed to the thigh, so that insulin absorption will be as predictable as possible.
- Do not exercise 60 to 90 minutes after injecting insulin, or when insulin action has reached its peak.
- Drink plenty of water before, during, and after exercise, as long as kidney disease is not a problem.

During exercise, have fruit juice or other rapidly absorbed carbohydrate fluids available. Exercise with a partner who understands what to do if you become hypoglycemic or lose consciousness. At the very least, carry identification that indicates you have diabetes and shows what medications you're taking to control it.

Recommended activities.   You may engage in any activity as long as you exercise with care. Regular aerobic activity for 20 to 30 minutes at a time is an important part of any treatment program. Low-impact aerobic activities such as walking, swimming, and cycling are preferred because they're less likely to bring on or aggravate leg and foot damage. Water exercises are beneficial (Figures 5.8–5.13). Weight training is generally safe. However, heavy straining may aggravate retinal damage, so consult with an ophthalmologist before you start.

Obesity

Obesity is the accumulation of excess body fat. As we get older, it is increasingly difficult to lose this extra weight.

Exercise precautions.   Avoid hot and humid conditions, since body fat provides extra insulation. Stay away from high-impact activities, because extra pounds place additional stress on the back, hips, knees, and feet.

Recommended activities.   Select low-impact activities such as walking, swimming, and cycling, which may be sustained comfortably for 40 to 60 minutes four or more days per week. In addition to a stretching and strengthening program for the water (Figures 5.8–5.13), try walking or jogging in waist-deep or chest-deep water.

LOWER-BACK PAIN AND SCIATICA

Pain in the lower back and aching or shooting discomfort down the side or back of the leg (sciatica) are among the most common physical problems seen in people over 40. Symptoms tend to come and go, and generally they don't reflect serious disease.

Lower-back pain and sciatica are usually brought on in one of two ways: (1) Muscles and ligaments that attach to the lower part of the spine (lumbar and sacral vertebrae) may suffer sprains and strains in the course of daily activities. Or (2) bulging disks, bone spurs, and tight muscles may press on the nerves that go down to the legs. Poor posture, work-related muscle strains, and structural imbalance due to curvature of the spine (scoliosis) may also lead to lower-back pain. Whatever the underlying cause, over 80 percent of lower-back pain is due to inadequate muscle strength and insufficient flexibility.

Exercise precautions.   Avoid high-impact activities such as jogging, high-impact aerobics, and sports that require jumping. The twisting required by serving in tennis and even playing golf may aggravate symptoms. If you lift weights, avoid heavy squats, since vertical forces are imposed directly on the lumbar spine.

Recommended activities.   In addition to regular aerobic exercise, the key to staying active is an ongoing stretching and strengthening program. This prevents symptoms in almost 90 percent of people.

Exercise for Sciatica

Stretching and strengthening.   Preferably, do conditioning exercises at least three times a week on the days when you aren't doing other activities. Lower-back exercises include mid- and lower-back and upper chest stretch (Figure 4.4), lower-back and buttock stretch (Figure 4.8), bent-knee sit-up (Figure 4.9), and the pelvic tilt (Figure 4.10). Rest for a few minutes, then do the complete body stretch (Figure 4.16). Continue with the two mid-back stretches (Figures 4.17 and 4.18), stomach crunches (Figure 4.20), and back-of-the-thigh (hamstring) stretch (Figure 4.25). You may do back extensions (Figure 4.21), but check with your doctor to make sure your back is strong enough.

Aerobic exercise.   For people with sciatica, bicycling, swimming (any strokes), and brisk walking on level ground provide excellent aerobic fitness. Alternate aerobic exercising with stretching and strengthening exercises on different days. If symptoms aren't present, integrate these activities into your regular exercise program.

Herniated Lumbar Disk

Lumbar disks can bulge out (herniate) between the vertebrae to press directly on nerve roots and cause disabling pain. This condition may bring on severe, acute pain, sometimes felt in the part of the body served by the nerve that is compressed. The most common herniations occur in the lower back, where the load-bearing forces are the greatest.

Exercise precautions.   Avoid weight lifting that puts pressure on the back. If you have a history of back problems such as herniated disk, or if you've had back surgery, check with your doctor before you start a vigorous activity program.

Recommended activities.   Follow the exercise program described above for sciatica.

NEUROLOGICAL DISORDERS

Some neurological disorders such as multiple sclerosis, stroke, and Parkinson's disease cause muscle weakness, affect coordination, and impair body movement. Other disorders, including epilepsy, may make exercise hazardous.

Movement Disorders and Muscle Weakness

If you have recovered from a stroke or polio, you may be left with some degree of weakness or even paralysis in the affected part of the body. Parkinson's disease causes tremor and stiffness, which usually impair both agility and coordination.

Exercise precautions.   Activities that require skill, agility, quickness, and balance (such as racquet sports, skiing, jogging, and cycling) may be difficult to perform. These activities also pose a risk of accidents or falls.

Benign familial tremors (mild shaking of hands that runs in families) that primarily affect the hands are common with increasing age. Although a tremor shouldn't limit your ability to exercise, your precision and coordination in skill sports such as bowling, tennis, or golf may be affected. Exercise is vital to maintain muscle function and aerobic fitness, but don't push to the point of fatigue or pain.

Recommended activities.   Continue with sports such as bowling, tennis, or golf by modifying your grip or arm motion. If your gait is altered or balance is affected in any way, the most appropriate choices are the basic fitness program (see chapter 4), light weight training using resistance machines, and walking or supervised water exercises (Figures 5.8–5.13). If you cycle, use a stationary bike or a three-wheeled bike.

Migraines and Other Headaches

Classic migraine headaches are characterized by visual symptoms, such as zigzag flashing lights, followed by severe, generally one-sided headaches.

Exercise precautions. Many people experience throbbing headaches when they're at altitudes above 8,000 feet. A small percentage of individuals have pounding head pain after sprinting or exercising to exhaustion. If you ordinarily have headaches and suddenly experience new or severe symptoms after physical activity, consult with a physician before resuming exercise.

Recommended activities. If you're feeling well, continue to do the activities of your choice.

Epilepsy and Seizures

An epileptic seizure consists of sudden electrical discharges in the brain. Seizures may bring on altered sensations, disturbances of movements, changes in perceptions or mood, and even complete loss of consciousness.

Exercise precautions. There's no particular sport that tends either to produce or to prevent seizures. However, the choice of activities depends on how well your seizures are under control. Generally speaking, if you've had no seizures for at least a year and your medications don't interfere with exercise (see chapter 6), there's no absolute prohibition on activity. If you are experiencing seizures, avoid activities and situations where a fall or even a brief lapse of consciousness might cause serious problems. Activities such as diving, climbing, vigorous cycling, and downhill skiing pose a risk. There's no clear consensus about the safety of swimming, but if you have an active seizure disorder, you shouldn't swim alone.

Recommended activities. You can participate in vigorous exercise. But before engaging in any activity, discuss it with your doctor.

PREGNANCY

Pregnancy places additional demands on circulation, and these demands increase as the fetus grows. Circulating hormones make the joints more flexible, and your center of gravity shifts as the fetus becomes larger. Both of these factors increase the risk of falling during exercise.

Exercise precautions. Aerobic and muscular fitness will help anyone deal with the physiological stresses of pregnancy and labor, but pregnancy is not an appropriate time to start a vigorous exercise program. If you should ever experience pain, bleeding, or any new symptoms or concerns, contact your obstetrician or registered nurse–midwife.

Recommended activities. If you're already fit, maintain your level of physical conditioning. If you're a jogger, continue jogging during pregnancy as long as it feels comfortable. Walking and low-impact, non-weight-bearing activities such as cycling and swimming are beneficial. If you wish to continue weight training, do it at a low intensity and without straining. You might want to do strengthening exercises for stomach, back, and legs. During the last three months of pregnancy, your capacity for exercise will diminish. The best guide is to exert yourself to a point where you can exercise comfortably and talk at the same time. Be careful to avoid overheating. As long as your pregnancy is normal, regular moderate exercise will not harm you or the fetus, or increase the risk of miscarriage.

RESPIRATORY DISORDERS

Mucus-producing cells line most of the upper breathing passages and parts of the lower respiratory tract. These tissues tend to swell and produce mucus when they're irritated, making it more difficult to get air through the passages.

Colds, Flu, and Acute Bronchitis

The common cold and other upper respiratory infections cause runny nose, sneezing, and scratchy throat. Infections such as bronchitis can also involve the upper lung passages.

Exercise precautions.   Vigorous and competitive activity is ill-advised when fever, muscle aches, loss of appetite, or chest cough and congestion are present. Fevers, sweats, chest pains, shortness of breath, and coughing up yellow, green, or brown mucus are all reasons to curtail activity and seek medical advice. Be especially cautious when you exercise outdoors. Cold air, wind, pollen, pollution, and dust may aggravate inflamed breathing passages.

Recommended activities.   If you have a cold or a viral flulike condition, you still can do moderate physical activity. If symptoms consist only of runny nose, sneezing, and scratchy throat, there's little risk. Use common sense.

Ear and Sinus Infections

Congestion and pressure in the middle-ear canals (eustachian tubes) and sinuses often accompany colds and allergies. Swimmers are susceptible to swimmer's ear (external otitis), the bacterial and fungal infection in the outer-ear canal. The ear opening may itch, swell, and ache, and there may be a yellowish or greenish discharge from the ear canal.

Exercise precautions.   If you have congestion in the head or pain in the cheeks or over the eyes, avoid underwater swimming and scuba diving. Decongestant medications may be beneficial for relieving the pressure that occurs in the closed sinus cavities and middle ear (see chapter 6). If you have swimmer's ear, prescription eardrops are usually required for prompt relief. To prevent swimmer's ear, wear earplugs and put a drop or two of a mixture of equal parts of isopropyl alcohol and vinegar into each ear canal after swimming.

Recommended activities.   Do your regular aerobic program as long as you feel comfortable and have taken proper precautions.

Hay Fever and Environmental Allergies

Up to 30 million Americans experience forms of allergic hay fever causing watery runny nose, itchy eyes, and nasal congestion.

Exercise precautions. Spasms of sneezing can be a problem when a short lapse of attention could cause an accident. Antihistamine medications used to control these symptoms may cause drowsiness as well (see chapter 6). Avoid underwater diving when you have head congestion.

Recommended activities. Continue your regular exercise program. Exercising indoors at those times of the year when seasonal pollens are a problem will help minimize symptoms.

Insect Allergies

An estimated one million Americans are at risk for allergic reactions to the venom of bees, yellow jackets, wasps, hornets, and fire ants. Although most stings and bites result only in localized pain and swelling, a minority of people experience hives, nausea, abdominal cramps, wheezing, clamminess, collapse of blood pressure, and possibly death.

Exercise precautions. Avoid golf, tennis, or other warm-weather outdoor activities if you're prone to life-threatening reactions. Carry a prescription insect-sting kit containing injectable epinephrine, and ask your doctor whether you need a series of injections to reduce your sensitivity.

Recommended activities. Any indoor activity and outdoor cool- or cold-weather activity is fine.

Asthma

The hallmarks of asthma are shortness of breath and wheezing caused by constricted breathing passages. An asthma attack may be triggered by specific allergies to ragweed, dust, animal dander, or pollens; by medications such as aspirin or ibuprofen; by smoke or chemical pollutants; or by physical irritants such as cold, dry air.

Exercise precautions. Aerobic exercise brings on symptoms in about 8 percent of the people who have asthma. Be cautious when scuba diving, because breathing compressed air may trigger an attack.

Recommended activities. The controlled breathing pattern of swimming (and the humidity at swimming pools) make it the best-tolerated aerobic activity. With jogging or other aerobic activity, warm up slowly for 10 minutes before you increase to your maximal effort. Wearing a surgical face mask (found in any drugstore) may prevent problems with outdoor aerobic exercise in cold, dry winter air. Ask your doctor if you should use inhaled medications prior to exercise.

Bronchial and Lung Problems

If you have shortness of breath from chronic bronchitis, emphysema, and other chronic lung diseases, you tend to expend more energy just to get air in and out of the lungs. The result is shortness of breath during activity.

Exercise precautions. Avoid exercising outdoors when pollution is heavy or the weather is hot and humid. High altitude may aggravate shortness of breath: Consider this when you plan trips and vacations.

Recommended activities. With emphysema and chronic bronchitis, weight training and aerobic activities such as walking and bicycling help build up stamina and increase respiratory capacity. When pollution or weather conditions worsen your symptoms, try "mall walking," or exercise in an indoor track or health club.

EYE PROBLEMS

Impaired Vision and Other Eye Problems

Common eye problems include dry eyes, retinal damage, cataracts, macular degeneration, and glaucoma.

Exercise precautions. For dry eyes, basic eye protection is important. Use goggles to protect the cornea from irritation when swimming, cycling, and skiing. Avoid sports such as racquetball or basketball, where direct eye trauma can occur. Most specialists advise patients with diabetic retinal damage to avoid the straining of heavy weight lifting and instead to use lighter weights and more repetitions. If visual symptoms or pain occurs with any exercise, consult your doctor.

Recommended activities. Follow the American College of Sports Medicine guidelines (see chapter 3). If you have retinal damage, cataracts, macular degeneration, or glaucoma, you can do almost anything as long as you use common sense. Do aerobic exercise with stationary equipment such as a treadmill, stationary bike, or step machine in a gym; if you jog, do it on a smooth track.

CHRONIC FATIGUE SYNDROME

There's no universal agreement on what causes chronic fatigue syndrome, but many physicians think that it may be the result of prior or ongoing viral infection.

Exercise precautions. Exercise may be a two-edged sword for chronic fatigue sufferers. It's important to stay as fit as possible, but even moderate physical activity may worsen symptoms. Be cautious with competitive activities that can demand a level of exertion beyond your capability.

Recommended activities. The best-tolerated activities are casual walking and swimming.

HIV INFECTION AND AIDS

People who are infected with HIV or who have AIDS should have a regular activity program.

Exercise precautions. If there are complicating infections that cause aches and fever, postpone activity unless you can perform it comfortably at a reduced intensity.

Recommended activities. Consult with your doctor about any exercise program you undertake.

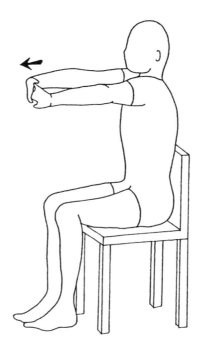

FIGURE 5.1 ARMS OUT Sit up straight with your feet flat on the floor. Interlock your fingers and invert your hands so that your palms are facing away. Stretch your arms out straight in front. Hold the stretch for a slow count of 15. Relax.

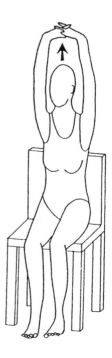

FIGURE 5.2   ARMS ABOVE   Sit up straight with your feet flat on the floor. Start by placing your hands on the top of your head. Interlock your fingers and invert your hands so your palms face the ceiling. Slowly reach your arms straight up over your head and stretch. Hold the stretch for a slow count to 15. Relax.

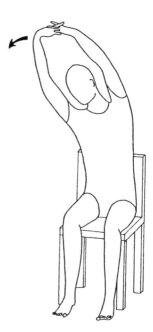

FIGURE 5.3   ARCH TO THE SIDE   Sit up straight with your feet flat on the floor. Interlock your fingers (without inverting your hands) to form an arch above your head. Slowly lean to the right and stretch. Hold for a slow count to 15. Then shift gradually to the left for a count of 15. Return your arms slowly to the center position. Bring your arms down and relax.

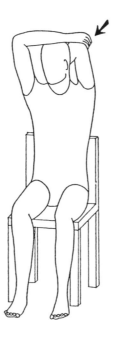

FIGURE 5.4 OUTER-SHOULDER (TRICEPS) STRETCH Sit up straight with your feet flat on the floor. Reach behind your head and touch the back of your right shoulder with your left hand. Use your right hand to push down on the left arm above the elbow. Hold for 10 seconds, then repeat with the opposite side. You'll feel the stretch on the upper part of the arm.

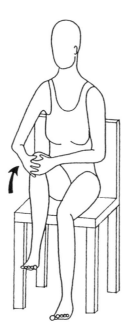

FIGURE 5.5 KNEES UP Sit up straight with your feet flat on the floor. Interlock your fingers over the front of the right leg just below the knee and slowly pull the leg up toward your chest—as high as it will go. Hold the stretch for a slow count to 15 and pull with your arms slightly bent. Slowly, let the leg down and relax. Repeat with the other side.

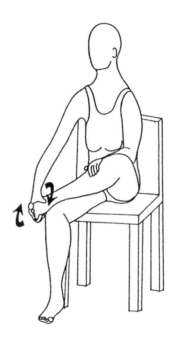

FIGURE 5.6 ANKLE LIFT AND TURN Sit up straight with your feet flat on the floor. Lift your left ankle and rest it on the top of your right knee. Grasp your foot and rotate the ankle clockwise five times, then rotate counterclockwise five times. Release. Repeat with the other leg.

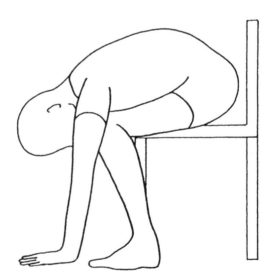

FIGURE 5.7 REACH TO THE FLOOR Sit up straight with your feet flat on the floor. Slowly bend forward and down. Touch the floor with the palms of your hands in front of your feet. Hold the stretch for a slow count to 15. Gradually return to an upright position.

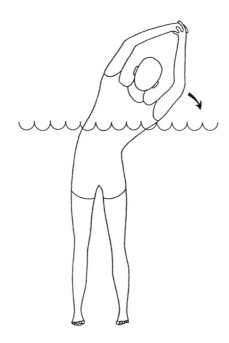

FIGURE 5.8   AQUA SIDE STRETCH   Stand in water up to your chest. Interlock your fingers (without inverting your hands) to form an arch above your head. Slowly lean to the left and stretch. Hold for a slow count to 15. Return your arms to the center position. Bring your arms down and relax. Repeat on the other side.

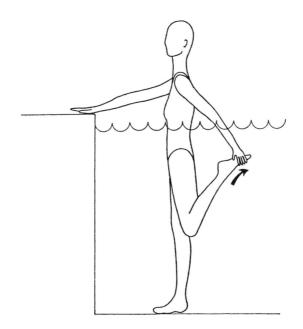

FIGURE 5.9   AQUA LEG (QUADRICEPS) STRETCH   Stand in water slightly above your waist and hold on to the side of the pool with your right hand. Grasp the front of the left foot and pull it back and up. Hold the stretch for a slow count to 15 or 20. Repeat with the other side.

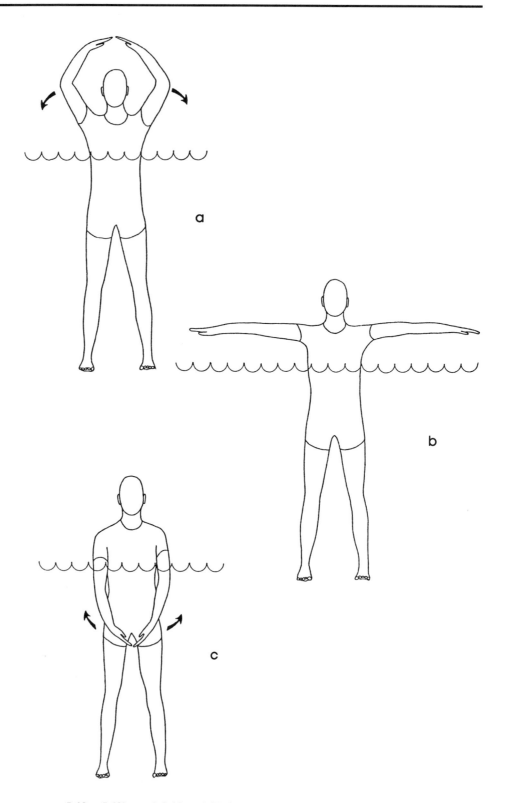

FIGURES 5.10a, 5.10b, and 5.10c AQUA ARM CIRCLES Stand in water up to your chest. Start with your arms overhead and your fingers touching. Slowly bring your arms out to the side and down through the water to touch your fingers underwater. Move your arms back up, out, and overhead. Repeat the full cycle 10 times.

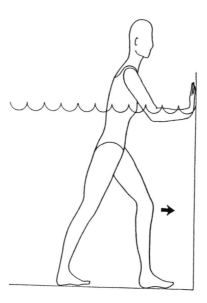

FIGURE 5.11   AQUA CALF AND HEEL STRETCH   Stand in water chest-deep with your arms stretched holding the side of the pool. Place your left foot flat on the bottom of the pool about six to eight inches from the side. Keep your right foot flat with your right leg extended behind you. Keep your feet flat at all times. While keeping the right leg straight, bend your left knee closer to the wall. Hold the stretch for a count to 15. Repeat with the opposite leg. Relax.

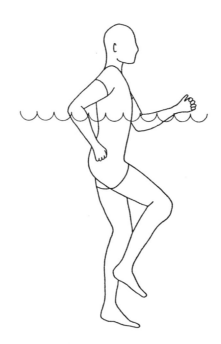

FIGURE 5.12   THE WATER MARCH   Standing in chest-deep water, either march in place or across the width of the pool. Continue for 60 seconds. Bend and move your arms naturally for balance.

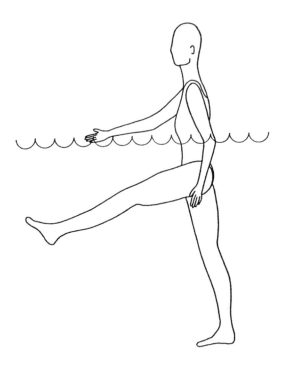

FIGURE 5.13   THE AQUA "GOOSE STEP"   In chest-deep water, do a "goose step" walk, keeping the knees straight. Walk slowly across the width of the pool. Continue for 60 seconds.

6

MIXING
EXERCISE AND MEDICATIONS

Every day millions of Americans take prescription drugs to treat acute or chronic medical conditions. An even greater number of people take nonprescription medications for aches, pains, heartburn, nasal congestion, and other common problems. Prescription drugs and over-the-counter medications—as well as substances such as caffeine, alcohol, and nicotine—may directly affect your ability to exercise.

This chapter provides an overview only, and shouldn't be used as the basis for altering a dosage or terminating any medication. Since each person's medical profile is unique, specific information about certain medications may not be directly applicable to your own situation. Address any questions you have about a particular drug directly to your physician.

MEDICATIONS AND EXERCISE—HOW THEY INTERACT

Many drugs produce more than one specific effect in your body. When any particular drug action inhibits or arrests your medical problem, relieves symptoms, or improves your function, that action is *therapeutic*. If a medication also produces discomfort or diminishes your body's performance or function, then the unwanted result is a *side effect*. Depending on the circumstances, the same drug actions may be therapeutic for one person and have undesirable side effects for another.

A good example of this complex relationship is the drug propranolol (*Inderal*), a beta-blocker. Propranolol slows the heart rate, decreases the forcefulness of heart pumping, and inhibits dilation of certain arteries. For someone who has coronary artery disease and angina pains on exertion, propranolol allows that person to achieve a higher workload before symptoms occur during aerobic activities such as cycling or brisk walking. In this case, holding down the heart rate and holding back the force of the heartbeat produce a therapeutic effect.

The actions of propranolol also lower blood pressure, and this drug is useful in the treatment of hypertension. For the person who has only high blood pressure and no chest pain on exertion, propranolol's effects on the heart rate and heart contraction decrease the maximum amount of effort that person can achieve. This may pose a problem if you combine propranolol with a vigorous activity such as competitive singles tennis. In this case, the medication can make you feel sluggish and affect your game. If you mix propranolol with a less strenuous sport, such as golf (which requires skill and a steady hand), then the slowing-down actions of propranolol are beneficial. In fact, propranolol use is banned during Olympic archery and target-shooting competition.

Activity itself can cause problems with medications, depending on when and where you exercise. As discussed earlier, vigorous activity slows stomach emptying. Therefore, medications taken too close to exercise periods may not be emptied from the stomach or absorbed from the intestinal tract. If they are not taken far enough in advance of exercise, drugs such as aspirin, ibuprofen, and other anti-inflammatory medications sit in the stomach. This causes irritation (gastritis) and possibly bleeding.

Where you exercise is the key element with skin rashes caused by exposure to ultraviolet light (photosensitivity). Medications, including some diuretics and antibiotics, can photosensitize a person. Skin rashes and even blistering can occur after snow skiing and sailing, because of the excessive amount of reflected sunlight. You can prevent many of these reactions if you avoid prolonged and intense sun exposure. Try to exercise early or late in the day. If you're at risk for photosensitivity reactions and you can't avoid sun exposure, wear a hat and cover up as much as possible. Use a sunscreen rated at SPF 15 or higher.

What This Means for You

Be cautious when you combine exercise with use of any drug or medication. While the instructions on the container and package insert provide a wealth of information, much of this information can be so sweeping and general that it's hard to tell whether it applies to your situation. The best source of guidance is your physician, and the answers to a few simple questions may be all you need.

When you're taking medication, or you want to know how nonprescription drugs or other substances interact with exercise, ask your doctor or pharmacist the following questions:

- How will this drug affect my exercising?
- Do I need to change my activity program in any way while I'm taking the drug?
- When should I take the medication in relation to when I exercise?
- Are there any precautions I should take or possible reactions I should be aware of?

If you have a specific concern about a medication that is prompted by information on the container or package insert, ask whether it applies to your circumstances.

PAIN RELIEVERS

Some pain relievers (analgesics) work directly to suppress irritation in the tissues where the pain originates. These medications are often used to treat arthritis, tendinitis, and related conditions. Because of their general effects, they may enhance your ability to exercise. Other analgesics work in the brain to alter your perception of painful stimuli. These drugs may cause drowsiness and interfere with physical activity, increasing your risk of an accident or injury.

Acetaminophen, Aspirin, and Combinations

Acetaminophen and aspirin are the primary ingredients in most nonprescription pain relievers. In recent years, ibuprofen has become available as a nonprescription pain reliever (see "Nonsteroidal Anti-Inflammatory Drugs," below).

These medications don't interfere with activity, so you may exercise as usual.

ACETAMINOPHEN, ASPIRIN, AND COMBINATIONS

- acetaminophen (*Tylenol, Datril, Phenaphen*)
- acetaminophen + caffeine (*Aspirin-Free Excedrin*)
- acetaminophen + caffeine + aspirin (*Excedrin*)
- aspirin (*Bufferin, Ascriptin, Ecotrin*)

Narcotics and Narcotic Combinations

Narcotics provide effective pain relief primarily by acting on nerve centers in the brain. They're often combined with aspirin or acetaminophen to attack pain at its origin as well. Be extra careful when you take these drugs. They can cause drowsiness, affect your reaction time, alter your perceptions, and impair your judgment. Avoid activities such as diving, downhill skiing, cycling, and climbing.

NARCOTICS AND NARCOTIC COMBINATIONS

- acetaminophen + codeine (*Tylenol 3*)
- acetaminophen + hydrocodone (*Vicodin, Lortab*)
- acetaminophen + oxycodone (*Percocet, Tylox*)
- acetaminophen + propoxyphene (*Darvocet-N*)
- acetaminophen + butalbital + caffeine (*Fioricet*)
- aspirin + codeine (*Empirin 3*)
- aspirin + oxycodone (*Percodan*)
- aspirin + butalbital + caffeine (*Fiorinal*)
- fentanyl (*Duragesic* patch)
- hydromorphone (*Dilaudid*)
- levorphanol (*Levo-Dromoran*)
- meperidine (*Demerol*)
- pentazocine (*Talwin*)

Nonsteroidal Anti-inflammatory Drugs (NSAIDs) Used for Pain

NSAIDs (pronounced "enseds") are medications that suppress inflammation (similar to the actions of steroids) in damaged tissues. They are widely used for the treatment of arthritis and related conditions, and some of them are particularly effective for relieving pain. (See also discussion of NSAIDs on pages 89–90.)

ANTIBIOTICS

Generally, you can be as active as you wish when you take oral antibiotics, so long as exercise doesn't interfere with your underlying medical condition. Some antibiotics may upset your stomach, so take them well in advance of activity. When your doctor gives you the prescription, ask if you need to change your exercise program.

Cephalosporins

Cephalosporins are used to treat skin as well as sinus, throat, bronchial, and lung infections. This family of drugs may also be prescribed for the treatment of bladder infections and diverticulitis of the colon.

Cephalosporins do not affect your normal activity program.

CEPHALOSPORINS

- cefaclor (*Ceclor*)
- cefadroxil (*Duricef*)
- cefixime (*Suprax*)
- cefpodoxime (*vantin*)
- cefprozil (*Cefzil*)
- cefuroxime (*Ceftin*)
- cephalexin (*Keflex*)
- loracarbef (*Lorabid*)

Erythromycins

Erythromycins are used in the treatment of skin, throat, bronchial, and lung infections. They are especially important for people who are allergic to penicillins. Take erythromycins well in advance of activity to guarantee their absorption by the body and to prevent stomach irritation.

ERYTHROMYCINS

- azithromycin (*Zithromax*)
- clarithromycin (*Biaxin*)
- erythromycin (*E.E.S., ERYC*)

Penicillins

Penicillins have a wide range of uses, most commonly in skin, urinary, upper and lower respiratory infections, as well as in sexually transmitted diseases. If you're allergic to one member of the penicillin family, however, assume that you're allergic to the others. With penicillins, you can maintain your regular exercise schedule. Check with your doctor to see if the underlying infection imposes any limits on your activity.

PENICILLINS

- amoxicillin (*Amoxil, Augmentin*)
- ampicillin (*Omnipen, Polycillin*)
- bacampicillin (*Spectrobid*)
- dicloxacillin (*Dynapen*)
- nafcillin (*Unipen*)
- penicillin (*Betapen-VK*)

Quinolones

Quinolones are powerful drugs used primarily to treat infections involving the bladder (cystitis) and prostate (prostatitis). They are also used for certain types of bronchitis. Take these drugs well in advance of exercise. If you have a urinary infection, drink plenty of fluids and avoid dehydration.

QUINOLONES

- cinoxacin (*Cinobac*)
- ciproflaxacin (*Cipro*)
- enoxacin (*Penetrex*)
- lomefloxacin (*Maxaquin*)
- norfloxacin (*Noroxin*)
- ofloxacin (*Floxin*)

Sulfa Drugs

The sulfas are most often used to treat urinary and prostate infections, traveler's diarrhea, and certain bronchial and lung infections. You can exercise as usual when you take these medications, but keep up your fluid intake.

SULFA DRUGS

- sulfamethizole (*Thiosulfil*)
- sulfamethoxazole + trimethoprim (*Bactrim, Septra*)
- sulfisoxazole (*Gantrisin*)

Tetracyclines

Tetracyclines are commonly prescribed for respiratory infections and skin conditions such as acne and rosacea, as well as traveler's diarrhea and certain sexually transmitted diseases. Avoid direct and prolonged sun exposure. All of the tetracyclines—doxycycline in particular—may cause a sun-induced rash (photosensitivity).

TETRACYCLINES

- doxycycline (*Vibramycin, Doryx*)
- minocycline (*Minocin*)
- tetracycline (*Achromycin*)

Other Oral Antibiotics

Clindamycin is used to treat certain types of bronchitis and pneumonia. (Antibiotic-associated diarrhea is frequently reported with this medication.) Metronidazole is prescribed for intestinal and vaginal infections. Nitrofurantoin and trimethoprim are used for certain urinary tract infections.

Exercise as you wish when you take these medications.

ORAL ANTIBIOTICS

- clindamycin (*Cleocin*)
- metronidazole (*Flagyl*)
- nitrofurantoin (*Macrodantin*)
- trimethoprim (*Proloprim*)

Antifungal Medications

Some antifungal medications are taken as pills; others are used as creams applied directly on the skin or in the vagina. Limit sun exposure when you take griseofulvin because of possible photosensitivity reactions. Apply vaginal antifungal medications after activity or at bedtime.

ANTIFUNGAL MEDICATIONS

- clotrimazole [vaginal] (*Gyne-Lotrimin*)
- fluconazole (*Diflucan*)
- griseofulvin (*Fulvicin*)
- itraconazole (*Sporanox*)
- ketoconazole (*Nizoral*)
- miconazole [vaginal] (*Monistat*)
- nystatin (*Mycostatin*)
- terconazole [vaginal] (*Terazol*)

Antiviral Agents

Acyclovir is the most commonly prescribed antiviral agent. It's used to fight oral herpes (fever blisters), genital herpes, and shingles (herpes zoster). Most of the other antiviral agents are prescribed for serious illnesses, including AIDS-related infections.

If you're taking acyclovir to treat an oral herpes infection, avoid sun exposure. Sunlight doesn't interact with the medication, but it may aggravate the herpes. If you're taking any of these medications, check with your doctor to see if exercise poses any special risks because of your underlying medical condition.

ANTIVIRAL AGENTS

- acyclovir (*Zovirax*)
- foscarnet (*Foscavir*)

- interferon (*Roferon-A, Intron A, Alferon N*)
- zidovudine (*Retrovir, AZT*)

ANTICANCER DRUGS

When you take these medications, the primary concern is whether you need to modify your activity programs because of the underlying malignancy.

Hormones and Antihormones

This family of drugs includes medications that are used to treat breast and prostate cancers. You can exercise as usual when you take these medications, unless you're advised not to by your doctor.

HORMONES AND ANTIHORMONES

- chlorotrianisene (*TACE*)
- diethylstilbestrol (*Stilphostrol*)
- flutamide (*Eulexin*)
- leuprolide (*Lupron*)
- megestrol (*Megace*)
- tamoxifen (*Nolvadex*)

Antimetabolites, Cytotoxic Agents, and Others

These medications inhibit the growth and multiplication of blood cells. They are used to treat malignancies such as leukemia and lymphomas. Check with your doctor to see if your underlying medical condition places any restrictions on your activities.

ANTIMETABOLITES AND CYTOTOXIC AGENTS

- busulfan (*Myleran*)
- chlorambucil (*Leukeran*)
- cyclophosphamide (*Cytoxan*)
- methotrexate (*Rheumatrex*)

ANTICOAGULANTS

Anticlotting medications such as warfarin interefere with the production of certain blood-clotting proteins. Other medications inhibit the clumping of those cells (platelets) in the blood that initiate the clotting process. These medications are used to prevent clotting in coronary bypass grafts, damaged leg veins, and in nonbeating upper heart chambers (atrial fibrillation). Avoid activities that could produce bleeding or bruising related to previous accidents, trauma, or severe impact. If you take warfarin, check with your doctor before you engage in activities where there may be limited access to emergency medical care.

ANTICOAGULANTS AND BLOOD THINNERS

- aspirin (*Bufferin, Ecotrin*)
- dipyridamole (*Persantine*)
- ticlopidine (*Ticlid*)
- warfarin (*Coumadin*)

ANTIARTHRITIS DRUGS

Anti-inflammatory medications may improve exercise function by relieving the irritations of tendinitis, bursitis, and arthritis. Whether you should exercise while you are taking these drugs depends more on your underlying medical condition than on the medications themselves.

Nonsteroidal Anti-inflammatory Drugs (NSAIDs)

The noncortisone anti-inflammatory drugs inhibit swelling, heat, pain, inflammation, and loss of function at the site of an injury or irritation. Be cautious with sun exposure, however, because NSAIDs may cause a sun-induced rash. Take these drugs with food or with a full glass of water well in advance of exercise. If they aren't fully absorbed by the time you start activity, they may irritate the stomach.

NSAIDs

- diclofenac (*Voltaren*)
- diflunisal (*Dolobid*)
- etodolac (*Lodine*)
- fenoprofen (*Nalfon*)
- flurbiprofen (*Ansaid*)
- ibuprofen (*Advil, Medipren, Motrin, Nuprin, Rufen*)
- indomethacin (*Indocin*)
- ketoprofen (*Orudis*)

- ketorolac (*Toradol*)
- meclofenamate (*Meclomen*)
- nabumetone (*Relafen*)
- naproxen (*Anaprox, Naprosyn*)
- oxaprozin (*Daypro*)
- piroxicam (*Feldene*)
- sulindac (*Clinoril*)
- tolmetin (*Tolectin*)

Corticosteroids

Cortisone medications are taken orally to treat conditions such as asthma, arthritis, eczema, and allergic reactions. They may also be administered by injection directly into an area of joint, ligament, or tendon inflammation.

Short-term use (one week or less) of oral corticosteroids doesn't affect exercise performance or capability, but long-term use of these medications may lead to osteoporosis and muscle weakness. When injected into an inflamed joint or tendon, cortisone medications can relieve inflammation but may temporarily inhibit repair of structures in the joint.

CORTICOSTEROIDS

- cortisone (*Cortone*)
- dexamethasone (*Decadron, Hexadol*)
- hydrocortisone (*Hydrocortone*)
- hydrocortisone methylprednisolone (*Medrol*)
- prednisone (*Deltasone*)
- triamcinolone (*Aristocort, Kenalog*)

Other Antiarthritis Drugs

Other anti-inflammatory medications may be used to treat rheumatoid arthritis, protect transplanted kidneys, and control psoriasis.

Take the medication well in advance of activity. Find out from your doctor how active you can be without aggravating the underlying arthritic condition. The medications themselves shouldn't influence your exercise.

ANTIARTHRITIS DRUGS

- azathioprine (*Imuran*)
- gold salts (*Myochrysine* injection, *Ridaura*)
- hydroxychloroquine (*Plaquenil*)
- methotrexate (*Rheumatrex*)
- penicillamine (*Cupramine*)

ASTHMA PREPARATIONS

Generally, lessening asthma symptoms enhances exercise capability, especially as it relates to aerobic performance.

Oral Medications

Oral asthma medications are absorbed into your system and may affect heart rate and keep you from sleeping. Some are related to amphetamines, and others to caffeine. These medications can make you feel jittery and shaky, which could impair your performance in deliberate activities such as shooting, archery, bowling, or golf.

ORAL ASTHMA MEDICATIONS

- albuterol (*Proventil, Ventolin*)
- metaproterenol (*Alupent, Metaprel*)
- terbutaline (*Brethine, Bricanyl*)
- theophylline (*Slophyllin, Theo-Dur, Uniphyl*)

Inhaled Preparations

Inhaled asthma medications open constricted breathing passages directly, and they may be absorbed into your system to some extent. Like their pill forms, these inhaled bronchodilators may cause jitteriness and impair skill in activities that require a steady hand.

INHALED ASTHMA MEDICATIONS

- albuterol (*Proventil, Ventolin*)
- bitolterol (*Tornalate*)

- epinephrine (*Primatene*)
- isoetharine (*Bronkometer, Bronkosol*)
- isoproterenol (*Isuprel*)
- metaproterenol (*Alupent, Metaprel*)
- pirbuterol (*Maxair*)
- terbutaline (*Brethaire*)

Other inhaled asthma medications fight inflammation and swelling in the breathing passages. These medications don't require special precautions with exercise.

INHALED ASTHMA MEDICATIONS

- beclomethasone (*Beclovent, Vanceril*)
- cromolyn (*Intal*)
- dexamethasone (*Decadron*)
- flunisolide (*AeroBid*)
- ipratropium (*Atrovent*)
- triamcinolone (*Azmacort*)

HEART MEDICATIONS

Cardiovascular drugs treat chest pain, heart attack, hypertension, and heart rhythm disorders, as well as blood vessel and blood flow problems. How a particular drug interacts with exercise depends primarily on your underlying medical condition. For this reason, consult with your physician if any exercise-related question or problem arises.

Angina and Coronary Artery Preparations

Angina pectoris is chest pain that occurs when the heart muscle's demand for oxygen exceeds the supply. Most often, angina is caused by coronary artery disease, and for a medication to be effective, it must either increase the amount of blood flowing to the heart muscle or reduce the amount of work the heart must perform. For people who have coronary artery disease, almost any of the antiangina medications improves exercise tolerance and stamina.

Beta-blocking drugs. Beta-blockers generally slow the heart rate and tone down the heart's beating. These drugs work primarily by reducing the heart's demand for blood and oxygen. Since these medications may inhibit the opening (dilation) of both bronchial passages in the lungs and blood vessels in the legs, they can cause pain or cramping in the legs as well as produce signs of asthma or wheezing. Beta-blockers also make some people feel tired or sluggish. Bring any exercise-related questions to your doctor's attention.

BETA-BLOCKERS

- atenolol (*Tenormin*)
- betaxolol (*Kerlone*)
- carteolol (*Cartrol*)
- metoprolol (*Lopressor, Toprol*)
- nadolol (*Corgard*)
- penbutolol (*Levatol*)
- propranolol (*Inderal*)
- timolol (*Blocadren*)

Calcium channel-blocking drugs. The calcium channel blockers primarily open up constricted blood vessels. There are no special concerns with exercise if you are taking these medications. (See "Calcium Channel Blockers" for specific drugs.)

Nitrates. Nitrate medications dilate narrowed blood vessels. They are so effective that you may develop a pounding headache shortly after you take one of these drugs. Nitrates generally don't interfere with exercise. In fact, many physicians prescribe them to be taken shortly before activity because they prevent exercise-induced angina (chest pain).

NITRATES

- isosorbide dinitrate (*Isordil, Sorbitrate*)
- isosorbide mononitrate (*Ismo*)
- nitroglycerin (*Nitrostat, Nitro-Bid, Nitro-Dur, Transderm-Nitro*)
- pentaerythritol tetranitrate (*Peritrate*)

Antihypertension Medications

Many of the drugs used to treat heart problems also play an important role in controlling elevated blood pressure. There is, however, a wide variation in how people respond to different blood pressure–lowering drugs.

Diuretics. Diuretics lower blood pressure by acting on the kidneys directly to promote the loss of sodium and water. The immediate result can be dehydration. Diuretics also cause potassium loss, which may produce muscle cramps and weakness. Drink plenty of fluids and eat potassium-rich foods such as bananas, raisins, and most dried fruits, when you exercise. This is especially important in warm weather. Combining hydrochlorothiazide with aldactone, triamterene, or amiloride helps minimize potassium loss, but for some people this still isn't enough. Also, hydrochlorothiazide is the diuretic most commonly associated with photosensitivity reactions, so be careful of sun exposure.

DIURETICS

- bumetanide (*Bumex*)
- chlorothiazide (*Diuril*)
- furosemide (*Lasix*)
- hydrochlorothiazide (*Esidrix, HydroDIURIL*)
- hydrochlorothiazide + aldactone (*Aldactazide*)
- hydrochlorothiazide + triamterene (*Dyazide, Maxzide*)
- hydrochlorothiazide + amiloride (*Moduretic*)
- indapamide (*Lozol*)
- methyclothiazide (*Enduron*)
- metolazone (*Diulo, Zaroxolyn*)

Beta-blocking drugs.   Beta-blockers slow the heart rate and decrease the forcefulness of heart pumping. They lower blood pressure primarily by decreasing the amount of blood pumped by the heart.

Beta-blockers may reduce stamina and decrease the amount of aerobic exercise you can perform. Muscle fatigue is a common side effect. Be alert for wheezing or shortness of breath if you have underlying lung disease. Watch for activity-induced calf cramps, which are caused by diminished blood flow to the legs. Also be careful if you're exercising in hot weather: Beta-blockers may interfere with blood flow to the skin and promote overheating.

BETA-BLOCKERS

- acebutolol (*Sectral*)
- atenolol (*Tenormin*)
- bisoprolol (*Zebeta*)
- labetolol (*Normodyne, Trandate*)
- metoprolol (*Lopressor, Toprol*)
- nadolol (*Corgard*)
- pindolol (*Visken*)
- propranolol (*Inderal*)
- timolol (*Blocadren*)

ACE inhibitors. Angiotensin-converting enzyme (ACE) inhibitors lower blood pressure by allowing blood vessels to open up. The ACE inhibitors are excellent choices for the active person who has high blood pressure. They do not interfere with maximal exercise capacity, and they're seldom associated with tiredness or fatigue.

ACE INHIBITORS

- benazepril (*Lotensin*)
- captopril (*Capoten*)
- enalapril (*Vasotec*)
- fosinopril (*Monopril*)
- lisinopril (*Prinivil, Zestril*)
- quinapril (*Accupril*)
- ramipril (*Altace*)

Alpha-blocking drugs. Alpha-blockers lower blood pressure by opening up narrowed blood vessels.

If you become dehydrated during exercise, you may feel light-headed. Otherwise, these medications don't interfere with exercise performance or capability.

ALPHA-BLOCKERS

- doxazosin (*Cardura*)
- prazosin (*Minipress*)
- terazosin (*Hytrin*)

Calcium channel-blocking drugs. These medications lower blood pressure by opening up blood vessels throughout the body.

None of these drugs interferes with exercise.

CALCIUM CHANNEL BLOCKERS

- amlodipine (*Norvasc*)
- diltiazem (*Cardizem, Dilacor*)
- felodipine (*Plendil*)

> - isradipine (*DynaCirc*)
> - nicardipine (*Cardene*)
> - nifedipine (*Procardia, Adalat*)
> - nimodipine (*Nimotop*)
> - verapamil (*Calan, Isoptin, Verelan*)

Miscellaneous drugs for high blood pressure. Some blood pressure medications don't fall into one of the families already listed. Clonidine and guanfacine may cause tiredness or drowsiness, so be cautious with exercises or activities that require quick reaction time or a high degree of skill.

OTHER HIGH BLOOD PRESSURE MEDICATIONS

> - clonidine (*Catapres*)
> - guanfacine (*Tenex*)
> - hydralazine (*Apresoline*)

Medications for Heart Failure

Two types of medications are used to treat heart failure. ACE inhibitors and diuretics (see earlier sections) work indirectly to reduce the amount of pumping the heart must do; digoxin (*Lanoxin, Lanoxicap*) acts directly on the heart muscle to augment its pumping ability.

Any drug that improves heart pumping also enhances exercise capability. Check with your doctor about the advisability of exercise as well as possible interactions between physical activity and medications.

Heart Rhythm Medications

If you are taking any medication to control your heart rhythm, check with your doctor about possible interactions between physical activity and your medications.

HEART RHYTHM MEDICATIONS

> - amiodarone (*Cordarone*)
> - beta-blockers: see discussion on pages 92–93, 94
> - calcium channel blockers: see discussion on pages 93, 95
> - digoxin (*Lanoxin*)
> - disopyramide (*Norpace*)

- encainide (*Enkaid*)
- flecainide (*Tambocor*)
- mexiletine (*Mexitil*)
- moricizine (*Ethmozine*)
- quinidine (*Cardioquin, Quinaglute, Quinidex*)
- procainamide (*Procan, Pronestyl*)
- propafenone (*Rhythmol*)
- tocainide (*Tonocard*)

CHOLESTEROL-LOWERING MEDICATIONS

Different drugs can reduce cholesterol and triglyceride levels, and therefore inhibit cholesterol plaque formation in the arteries. If you take cholestyramine, do so only after you exercise, since it may cause bloating and abdominal discomfort during vigorous activity. Take nicotinic acid with food, at least several hours before you exercise. These medications shouldn't affect your exercise capability or performance.

CHOLESTEROL-LOWERING MEDICATIONS

- cholestyramine (*Questran*)
- clofibrate (*Atromid*)
- gemfibrozil (*Lopid*)
- lovastatin (*Mevacor*)
- nicotinic acid (niacin, *Nicobid*)
- pravastatin (*Pravachol*)
- probucol (*Lorelco*)
- simvastatin (*Zocor*)

COLD, COUGH, AND ALLERGY PREPARATIONS

More than 30 million Americans each year use antihistamines, decongestants, or combinations of these drugs to relieve allergy and cold symptoms. In many cases, over-the-counter medications are just as potent as (and sometimes identical to) the drugs that require a prescription.

Antihistamines

Antihistamines block the effects of histamine, a chemical released in body tissues during allergic reactions and some infections. Antihistamines help to reduce or prevent the congestion, swelling, and itching caused by histamine.

ANTIHISTAMINES

- astemizole (*Hismanal*)
- brompheniramine (*Dimetane*)
- chlorpheniramine (*Chlor-Trimeton*)
- clemastine (*Tavist*)
- diphenhydramine (*Benadryl*)
- loratadine (*Claritin*)
- terfenadine (*Seldane*)
- tripelennamine (*PBZ*)

Be very careful when you take antihistamine preparations. Antihistamines can cause sedation and drowsiness, and even if you do not feel drowsy, most antihistamines impair coordination, judgment, and overall performance. Diphenhydramine is so sedating that it is often sold as a nonprescription sleeping medication. Avoid antihistamines when you dive, because they may alter your judgment and perception of time, a dangerous combination in deep water. Cycling, skiing, or even using a stair climber may be dangerous because antihistamines tend to slow your reaction time. Mental impairment persists even after the sense of drowsiness resolves, and this may diminish your performance in skill sports by affecting both your coordination and your ability to stay "focused." The newer second-generation antihistamines—astemizole, loratadine, and terfenadine—do not tend to cause drowsiness or impair performance, but it's best to be cautious with these preparations as well.

Decongestants

Decongestants, especially in large doses, can cause an accelerated heart rate and shakiness. This can affect golf and archery, both of which require steady hands. Weight lifters should be aware that decongestants may bring on dangerously high blood pressure. Decongestant nasal sprays may dry the nasal membranes to such an extent that nosebleeds occur, especially during exercise in low humidity, in the cold, and at high altitudes.

DECONGESTANTS

- oxymetazoline (*Afrin*)
- phenylephrine (*Neo-Synephrine, Dristan Nasal Spray*)
- phenylpropanolamine (*Entex*)
- pseudoephedrine (*Sudafed, Afrin* tablets)

Combinations of Antihistamine and Decongestant

Take the same precautions when you use a combination antihistamine and decongestant as when you take either one alone. The stimulating actions of the decongestant may balance the sedative effects of the antihistamine, but the net effect of the medication is difficult to predict for any given person.

Narcotic Cough Suppressants

Do not combine these medications with activities that require quick judgment, agility, and split-second reaction. Although dextromethorphan is the safest of the three anticough medications, such drugs are often combined with antihistamines, which add to the potential for sedation and functional impairment.

NARCOTIC COUGH SUPPRESSANTS

- codeine (*Robitussin A-C*)
- dextromethorphan (*Robitussin DM*)
- hydrocodone (*Hycodan, Hycomine*)

MEDICATIONS FOR SKIN DISORDERS

Dermatological Creams and Lotions

Be on the lookout for photosensitivity reactions with fluorouracil, isotretinoin, and tretinoin, medications that are used to treat skin cancer and acne.

DERMATOLOGICAL MEDICATIONS

- fluorouracil (*Efudex*)
- isotretinoin (*Accutane* capsules)
- minoxidil (*Rogaine*)
- tretinoin (*Retin-A*)

Medications for Itching and Hives

All of these medications may cause drowsiness. They may slow reaction time and affect your performance in skill sports. Refrain from diving because your time sense and judgment may be impaired.

MEDICATIONS FOR ITCHING AND HIVES

- cyproheptadine (*Periactin*)
- diphenhydramine (*Benadryl*)
- hydroxyzine (*Atarax, Vistaril*)
- methdilazine (*Tacaryl*)
- trimeprazine (*Temaril*)

MEDICATIONS FOR DIABETES

The greatest concern about exercise and medications that lower blood sugar is the risk of developing low blood sugar, especially right after activity.

Insulin

If you need insulin injections to control blood sugar, ask your doctor about possibly adjusting your insulin dose before exercise. Also inquire about any special recommendations that relate to eating or drinking during activity. Don't drink alcoholic beverages after you exercise, because this may increase the risk of hypoglycemic (low blood sugar) reactions (sweating, palpitations, shakiness). Before exercising, it may be wise for you to inject insulin into the abdominal wall rather than the thigh. Leg exercise may hasten the absorption of insulin from the thigh, although there is no uniform agreement about this among diabetes specialists.

Oral Medications

Be especially careful if you're also taking a beta-blocker such as propranolol (*Inderal*). Beta-blockers mixed with these medications may aggravate a hypoglycemic reaction.

ORAL DIABETES MEDICATIONS

- chlorpropamide (*Diabinese*)
- glipizide (*Glucotrol*)
- glyburide (*DiaBeta, Glynase, Micronase*)
- tolazamide (*Tolinase*)
- tolbutamide (*Orinase*)

MEDICATIONS FOR STOMACH AND INTESTINAL DISORDERS

Antacids

All antacids can lead to kidney-stone formation, so avoid dehydration during activity. Magnesium-containing antacids may cause diarrhea, possibly aggravating "runners' trots."

ANTACIDS

- calcium carbonate (*Tums*)
- calcium carbonate + aluminum hydroxide (*Di-Gel*)
- magaldrate (*Riopan*)
- magnesium + aluminum hydroxide (*Maalox, Mylanta*)

Medications for Ulcers and Hyperacidity

Acid distress and heartburn may occur with exercise. When this is the case, antiulcer medications may enhance exercise capability.

Medications to reduce stomach acid. Certain members of the antihistamine family are effective for reducing the amount of acid produced by cells lining the stomach. These medications are safe to use with exercise. On rare occasions, cimetidine (*Tagamet*) causes drowsiness or confusion, which could affect safety during diving, cycling, climbing, and skiing.

MEDICATIONS THAT REDUCE STOMACH ACID

- cimetidine (*Tagamet*)
- famotidine (*Pepcid*)
- nizatidine (*Axid*)
- omeprazole (*Prilosec*)
- ranitidine (*Zantac*)

Other medications for the stomach. Neither misoprostol nor sucralfate should affect physical activity. Metoclopramide may cause drowsiness and interfere with those activities that require sound judgment, quickness, or agility.

STOMACH MEDICATIONS

- cisapride (*Propulsid*)
- metoclopramide (*Reglan*)
- misoprostol (*Cytotec*)
- sucralfate (*Carafate*)

Nausea Medications

Be cautious if you take any nausea medications prior to exercise. In particular, avoid diving if you are using these medications for seasickness. These drugs can affect the temperature-regulating area of the brain and inhibit your ability to adjust to both hot and cold environments. They may alter your sense of time, impair your judgment, and affect your reaction time and coordination. Your performance may suffer in skill sports and in those activities that require agility and quick reactions.

NAUSEA MEDICATIONS

- cyclizine (*Marezine*)
- dimenhydrinate (*Dramamine*)
- meclizine (*Antivert, Bonine*)
- prochlorperazine (*Compazine*)
- promethazine (*Phenergan*)
- scopolamine patch (*Transderm Scōp*)
- trimethobenzamide (*Tigan*)

Digestive Enzymes

These substances help the body break down proteins, fats, and carbohydrates so they can be absorbed by the intestines. These medications have no adverse effects on your exercise capability. In fact, by aiding the absorption of food from the intestines, they can enhance your comfort during activity.

DIGESTIVE ENZYMES

- pancreatin (*Donnazyme, Entozyme*)
- pepsin (*Donnazyme, Entozyme, Pancrease, Lipase*)

Fiber Supplements

If you find that bulk or fiber preparations increase abdominal cramping, bloating, and flatulence when you exercise, lower the dosage and inform your doctor.

FIBER SUPPLEMENTS

- methylcellulose (*Citrucel*)
- psyllium (*Effer-Syllium, Fiberall, Metamucil, Perdiem*)

Antispasmodics

With any of the antispasmodics, avoid activities that require good judgment, agility, and fast reactions. These medications, particularly those that contain phenobarbital or chlordiazepoxide (*Librium*), may impair your reactions and make your drowsy. Be especially careful in hot weather, because the same drug effects that prevent spasms also impair sweating and possibly lead to heat-stroke.

ANTISPASMODICS

- clidinium + chlordiazepoxide (*Librax*)
- dicyclomine (*Bentyl*)
- hyoscyamine (*Levsin, Levsinex*)
- hyoscyamine + phenobarbital (*Donnatal*)
- propantheline (*Pro-Banthīne*)

Diarrhea Medications

All of these medications may impair your judgment or cause drowsiness. Avoid activities such as diving, where awareness of time and alertness are required.

DIARRHEA MEDICATIONS

- diphenoxylate (*Lomotil*)
- loperamide (*Imodium*)
- tincture of opium (*Donnagel-PG*, paregoric)

HORMONES

Hormones, when taken to correct a deficiency in your body's own production of hormones, should enhance your exercise capability as well as overall physical function.

Androgens

There are no adverse effects on exercise when you take replacement doses of male hormones. Some body builders take testosterone or other steroids, but these can produce dangerous side effects and should be avoided unless prescribed by a physician for a medical reason.

ANDROGENS

- fluoxymesterone (*Halotestin*)

Estrogens and Progestogens

The body's production of female hormones diminishes with menopause. You may exercise as usual when taking replacement doses of hormones.

You may also exercise as usual when you're taking replacement doses of progestogens, unless your doctor advises you otherwise.

ESTROGENS AND PROGESTOGENS

- conjugated estrogens (*Premarin*)
- diethylstilbestrol
- estradiol (*Estrace, Estraderm*)
- estropipate (*Ogen*)
- ethinyl estradiol (*Estinyl*)
- medroxyprogesterone (*Depo-Provera, Provera*)
- norethindrone (*Aygestin*)
- quinestrol (*Estrovis*)

Thyroid Preparations

You don't have to take any special precautions when you take replacement doses of thyroid medication.

THYROID PREPARATIONS

- dessicated thyroid, USP
- -thyroxine (*Synthroid, Levothroid*)
- -triiodothyronine (*Cytomel*)

MUSCLE RELAXANTS AND MEDICATIONS FOR NEUROLOGICAL DISORDERS

Migraine Preparations

Blood vessels throughout the body can be affected by these medications. When the blood vessels in the skin are prevented from opening, you will become more susceptible to frostbite. In hot, humid weather, you're more likely to overheat during exercise.

MIGRAINE MEDICATIONS

- ergotamine (*Cafergot, Ergostat*)
- isometheptene (*Midrin*)
- sumatriptan (*Imitrex* injection)

Medications for Parkinson's Disease

Consult with your physician before starting an exercise program. A fall in blood pressure when you stand up (a common effect of Parkinson's disease) can worsen if you take carbidopa and levodopa.

MEDICATIONS FOR PARKINSON'S DISEASE

- biperiden (*Akineton*)
- bromocriptine (*Parlodel*)
- carbidopa-levodopa (*Sinemet*)
- levodopa (*Larodopa*)
- pergolide (*Permax*)
- selegiline (*Eldepryl*)

Seizure Medications

All seizure medications may make you drowsy. Take care with activities such as skiing, cycling, riding, diving, and swimming.

SEIZURE MEDICATIONS

- carbamazepine (*Tegretol*)
- clonazepam (*Klonopin*)
- divalproex (*Depakote*)
- ethosuximide (*Zarontin*)
- phenobarbital
- phenytoin (*Dilantin*)
- primidone (*Mysoline*)
- valproic acid (*Depakene*)

Muscle Relaxants

These medications may impair judgment and cause drowsiness. Avoid skill sports and activities such as diving, skiing, climbing, and cycling; all require agility, quick reactions, and a clear mind.

MUSCLE RELAXANTS

- carisoprodol (*Soma*)
- chlorzoxazone (*Parafon*)
- cyclobenzaprine (*Flexeril*)
- diazepam (*Valium*)
- methocarbamol (*Robaxin*)

OSTEOPOROSIS MEDICATIONS

Calcium supplements provide the raw material for bones, whereas etidronate promotes the utilization of calcium in the bone-rebuilding process. By increasing bone mass, these medications decrease the risk of fractures.

OSTEOPOROSIS MEDICATIONS

* calcium (*Dical-D, Os-Cal, Tums*)
* etidronate (*Didronel*)

MEDICATIONS FOR DEPRESSION, ANXIETY, AND PSYCHOSIS

Most medications that control anxiety and treat depression have the potential to impair judgment, affect coordination, and cause drowsiness.

Antianxiety Medications

With the exception of buspirone, all of these medications produce an effect similar to that of alcohol. Avoid cycling, skiing, climbing, and any other activity that requires fast reactions.

ANTIANXIETY MEDICATIONS

* alprazolam (*Xanax*)
* buspirone (*BuSpar*)
* chlordiazepoxide (*Librium*)
* clorazepate (*Tranxene*)
* diazepam (*Valium*)
* lorazepam (*Ativan*)
* meprobamate (*Miltown*)
* oxazepam (*Serax*)
* prazepam (*Centrax*)

Antidepressants

Antidepressants alter the chemical balance in the brain tissue in order to help elevate mood.

Tricyclic antidepressants. Any of these medications may make you drowsy. They may also cause low blood pressure and dizziness when you stand up, an effect that is aggravated by dehydration.

TRICYCLIC ANTIDEPRESSANTS

- amitriptyline (*Elavil, Endep*)
- amitriptyline + chlordiazepoxide (*Limbitrol*)
- amitriptyline + perphenazine (*Etrafon, Triavil*)
- amoxapine (*Asendin*)
- clomipramine (*Anafranil*)
- doxepin (*Sinequan*)
- imipramine (*Tofranil*)
- maprotiline (*Ludiomil*)
- nortriptyline (*Pamelor*)
- protriptyline (*Vivactil*)
- trazodone (*Desyrel*)
- trimipramine (*Surmontil*)

MAO inhibitors. Monoamine oxidase (MAO) inhibitors may themselves dramatically lower blood pressure. These medications also interact with tyramine-rich foods (e.g., cheddar cheese) and nonprescription cold medications, and may raise blood pressure to alarmingly high levels. Check with your doctor before you start to exercise.

MAO INHIBITORS

- isocarboxazid (*Marplan*)
- phenelzine (*Nardil*)
- tranylcypromine (*Parnate*)

Other antidepressants. These newer mood-elevating medications tend to produce far fewer side effects than do the tricyclic antidepressants. Generally, this group of drugs doesn't interfere with physical activity.

OTHER ANTIDEPRESSANTS

- bupropion (*Wellbutrin*)
- fluoxetine (*Prozac*)
- lithium (*Eskalith, Lithobid*)

* paroxetine (*Paxil*)
* sertraline (*Zoloft*)

Antipsychotics and Major Tranquilizing Medications

These medications may alter your ability to stay warm in the cold or stay cool in the heat. Moreover, they may cause drowsiness and impair your judgment. Consult with your doctor before you start an exercise program.

ANTIPSYCHOTICS

* chlorpromazine (*Thorazine*)
* chlorprothixene (*Taractan*)
* clozapine (*Clozaril*)
* fluphenazine (*Prolixin*)
* haloperidol (*Haldol*)
* loxapine (*Loxitane*)
* mesoridazine (*Serentil*)
* perphenazine (*Trilafon*)
* thioridazine (*Mellaril*)
* thiothixene (*Navane*)
* trifluoperazine (*Stelazine*)

Sleeping medications and sedatives Flurazepam is long-acting and may leave you with a "hangover." All of these drugs can interfere with activities that require concentration and quick reactions.

SEDATIVES

* estazolam (*ProSom*)
* flurazepam (*Dalmane*)
* quazepam (*Doral*)
* secobarbital (*Seconal*)
* temazepam (*Restoril*)
* triazolam (*Halcion*)
* zolpidem (*Ambien*)

MEDICATIONS FOR BLADDER AND KIDNEY DISORDERS

Urinary Bladder Antispasmodics

With any of the antispasmodics, avoid activities that require good judgment, agility, and fast reactions.

ANTISPASMODICS

- atropine + hyoscyamine (*Urised*)
- hyoscyamine (*Cystospaz-M*)
- oxybutynin (*Ditropan*)

Medications for Prostate Enlargment

There are no exercise precautions when you're taking finasteride. Prazosin and terazosin can cause dehydration, making you feel light-headed.

PROSTATE MEDICATIONS

- finasteride (*Proscar*)
- prazosin (*Minipress*)
- terazosin (*Hytrin*)

VITAMINS

Vitamin supplements do not appear to enhance exercise performance or increase endurance. Large doses of vitamin C (over 1,000 mg per day) may contribute to the risk of developing kidney stones. Drink plenty of fluids during physical activity. Large doses of vitamins A and D can be toxic over time.

NONMEDICINAL DRUGS

Nonmedicinal drugs and substances do not enhance exercise capability for the most part, and they are often the source of exercise-related problems and injuries.

Alcohol

Alcohol and exercise are not a good mix. Because alcohol impairs judgment, slows reaction time, and interferes with coordination, it plays a major role in diving accidents, drowning, skiing injuries, and deaths from exposure to the cold (hypothermia). Alcoholic beverages are terrible choices for fluid replacement. Taken prior to endurance activities, alcohol leads to dehydration and low blood sugar. When consumed immediately after exercise on an empty stomach, alcohol rapidly produces intoxicating effects.

Anabolic Steroids

The use of anabolic steroids in conjunction with a vigorous weight-training program will result in increases in muscle bulk and strength. But their use promotes hair growth and masculinization in women, decreased fertility, atherosclerosis, raises the risk of liver tumors, and may induce severe emotional and even psychotic reactions. Moreover, injecting steroids with shared needles could transfer hepatitis and AIDS viruses, as well as other blood-borne infections. The possession of most anabolic steroids is illegal in the United States.

Caffeine

For the vast majority of people, drinking moderate amounts of coffee, tea, or caffeinated soft drinks well in advance of exercise doesn't affect exercise capability. Those who are habituated to caffeine may feel more sluggish without it in the morning, but exercise performance is unlikely to suffer. If you consume caffeine just prior to exercise, it has the potential to cause irritability, tremor, nervousness, and irregular heart rhythms. This could affect your performance in skill sports where a steady hand is needed. Interestingly, vigorous aerobic exercise slows the elimination of caffeine from the body, possibly prolonging any adverse effects in people who are sensitive to the drug.

Tobacco

Tobacco impairs exercise performance because of two major toxins—carbon monoxide and nicotine. Carbon monoxide is absorbed from inhaled tobacco smoke, yours or someone else's. Nicotine is absorbed not only from smoke but also from oral smokeless tobacco through the cheek lining and from juice that is swallowed. Other sources of nicotine include the prescription nicotine gums and patches. Smokers have a reduced degree of endurance, which is directly related to how much they smoke. Carbon monoxide displaces oxygen from the blood, and it reduces the maximal effort you can sustain. Nonsmokers who live with people who smoke two packs daily inhale the equivalent of three cigarettes per day, enough to diminish exercise performance.

Nicotine is a potent constrictor of the arteries, diminishing blood flow to the skin surface (especially of the fingers and toes). This arterial constriction increases susceptibility to exposure and frostbite. Nicotine is eliminated from your body more slowly during high-intensity exercise, and this affects energy metabolism by lessening blood flow to the muscles. The result may be the faster onset of muscle fatigue and diminished exercise performance.

Recreational Drugs

The use of marijuana, cocaine, and amphetamines does not enhance performance. The intoxication and altered judgment produced by these substances may cause you to take risks that would otherwise be avoided.

7
COPING WITH INJURY

Many people tend to disregard aches and pains that occur during or after exercise. In the early stages of many injuries, it's sometimes difficult to ascertain if there's a real problem. To help you pinpoint a serious problem, ask yourself:

- When and how did the problem start?
- Does the injured area appear normal? Is there any localized tenderness, swelling, discoloration, or change in appearance?
- Is there any functional impairment? Do moving parts move normally?
- Do the symptoms occur at the beginning of activity, during activity, or after you stop?
- Has there been a recent change in your exercise program—frequency, intensity, or length of workouts?

It's helpful to record the answers on paper or in a log so that you can identify a more precise pattern of what you're experiencing.

TYPES OF INJURIES

Exercise-related injuries fall into two broad categories: First are the sudden sprains, strains, breaks, and tears when the cause is obvious. Second are the less obvious acute or chronic "wear-and-tear" injuries. With these overuse injuries, the precise cause may not only be unclear, but symptoms may actually improve temporarily when you exercise.

TREATING EXERCISE-RELATED INJURIES

Once you've recognized that there's an injury, follow these four principles:

1. Stop the activity that is causing the injury.
2. Minimize the tissue damage.
3. Strengthen and condition the affected parts of the body.
4. Reassess your exercise program in order to prevent future problems.

Self-help: The RICE Treatment

The acronym RICE is an effective way to remember the first-aid steps for treating most exercise-related injury. It stands for

> **R**est
> **I**ce
> **C**ompression
> **E**levation

First, *rest* by stopping the activity that has caused the injury. Use *ice* or frozen gel packs to reduce tissue damage and swelling, and to control pain and irritation that may immediately follow exercise. (A plastic bag filled with ice and water works very well. Place a towel or elastic bandage between the ice pack and skin.) Apply the ice for 10 to 15 minutes immediately after the injury, then use it 10 minutes on and 10 minutes off for the next two hours.

If the involved part of the body is swelling, apply *compression* by using an elastic wrap or bandage. Don't bandage it so tightly that the part of the body below the injury becomes cool or pale (cutting off circulation). *Elevate* the injured area as much as possible to reduce and prevent further swelling.

Most injuries begin to improve after 48 hours of RICE treatment. Agents such as aspirin or ibuprofen also help relieve pain and inflammation. Acetaminophen can decrease pain.

When to Seek Professional Help

Seek prompt professional medical attention anytime you

- are completely unable to use or move the injured area
- notice any change in the usual shape of an injured bone
- feel constant or unrelieved pain in the injured area
- notice bruising or swelling at a joint or over a bone, together with pain when you move or bear weight
- experience temporary loss of consciousness

Anytime you experience recurring or persistent exercise-associated pain, stiffness, or loss of function, see your physician first. A physiotherapist who specializes in sports medicine can be helpful.

SKIN INJURIES AND PROBLEMS

Abrasions

Causes and symptoms. Painful abrasions occur primarily with bicycling, football, hiking and climbing, jogging, roller skating and roller-blading, and tennis. One or more layers of skin may be scraped away, and the depth of the injury often varies in different parts of the wound.

Self-help. Clean the wound gently with soap and warm running water, then cleanse the area around the wound with an antiseptic such as rubbing (isopropyl) alcohol. Blot the area dry, and keep the damaged skin clean. Nonstick dressings are necessary only to protect the area from dirt or to prevent clothing from sticking to the skin. An antibiotic ointment is usually not needed unless the wound was particularly dirty. Wear protective clothing and equipment appropriate for your activity (gloves and long sleeves for cycling, elbow and knee pads for roller skating/blading).

Professional help. Seek medical help if you think that tendon, muscle, or bone surfaces are visible, if there's any embedded material that can't be easily removed, if the wound becomes more painful and pus is noted, or if the surrounding skin becomes red and painful.

Cuts and Lacerations

Causes and symptoms. Most activity-related lacerations aren't sharp cuts. Instead they tend to be a combination of crushing and tearing of tissue.

Self-help. First, control the bleeding. Apply pressure to the wound with a clean cloth or pad for at least three minutes, and elevate the injured area if possible. Clean the wound with soap, and use running water to wash out any dirt, sand, or other debris. If the injury is shallow and there's a flap of skin that's partially attached, put the piece of skin back in place. Use sterile strips or an adhesive "butterfly" tape to keep the edges of the wound together. Keep the injury as dry as possible, and apply nonstick sterile gauze or a bandage to keep the wound clean. To "air" the wound, the dressing may be removed at night, avoiding contact with bedclothes and linen, then reapplied in the morning after inspecting and gently cleansing around the wound.

Professional help. If the wound is more than one inch long or gapes open, see a physician. If the laceration is small but in a cosmetically sensitive area such as the face, you may want to consult a plastic surgeon.

Blisters

Causes and symptoms. The top layer of skin (epidermis) separates from the deeper layer (dermis), and clear fluid accumulates in between. The blood vessels and nerves are located in the dermis, and once the protective epidermis is lost, the remaining surface is raw and very sensitive.

Self-help. If the blister has already ruptured and the roof of it remains attached, leave it in place as long as the point of rupture is small. If the skin is tattered, you may trim it with a pair of sharp scissors. Clean the blister with either dilute hydrogen peroxide or warm soapy water. Use a nonstick bandage. Repeat this process several times daily until the blister heals. If the roof of the blister hasn't ruptured, puncture it with a sterilized needle to let the fluid out. Repeat the puncture up to three times within the first 24 hours after the blister appeared. Remember that each separate puncture requires another sterile needle or a newly resterilized pin.

Professional help. Contact your physician if the fluid becomes cloudy or bloody, or if redness, swelling, or pain develops around the blister site.

Calluses

Causes and symptoms. A callus is a thickening of the surface of the skin that forms in response to repeated friction. Discomfort arises when the callus presses on the underlying structures (the "stone in the shoe" effect).

Self-help. Use a pumice stone, nail file, or emery board to grind away the thickened skin. If gentle measures aren't effective, *under no circumstances try to remove a callus with a razor blade or knife.* Apply petroleum jelly to the callus before you exercise. This will help reduce friction and prevent further skin thickening.

Professional help. If you can't remove a callus on the foot with simple remedies, see a podiatrist.

Corns

Causes and symptoms. Corns represent thickening in the deepest layers of skin. They cause pain with direct pressure because of their location over bones.

Self-help. Over-the-counter solutions to remove corns are effective for reducing small corns. Small doughnut-type pads (sold in pharmacies) may provide protection from pressure that contributes to their formation. Unlike calluses that form on the surface of a toe or foot, corns develop where skin surfaces rub together. Never try to grind down a corn.

Professional help. If corns remain painful or if you are a diabetic, see a podiatrist.

Chafing

Causes and symptoms. Repeated rubbing wears away the surface layer of the skin, leaving the underlying layer raw and exposed. Common sites of chafing include the inner thighs (from cycling and running), under the arms (from jogging), and on the nipples of both men and women (from jogging and racquet sports). Chafing can be so painful that it becomes difficult to continue your activity. Fortunately, chafing is a superficial injury and it heals rapidly.

Self-help. Simply keep the skin clean and dry, and avoid further rubbing. Before you resume activity, coat the skin under the arms and on the thighs with petroleum jelly to reduce friction. To prevent painful irritation, women can wear a sports bra. Men can place an adhesive strip over the nipples.

Professional help. Unless infection is present, professional help isn't necessary.

TOE AND FRONT-FOOT INJURIES

Black Toenail

Causes and symptoms. Black toenail is usually a painless condition most often involving the second (and longest) toe. Chronic friction from bumping or rubbing against the end of the shoe may cause bleeding under the toenail. It's brought on by walking downhill and running, and by starting and stopping abruptly during racquet sports. If the toenail is loosened enough, it will fall off naturally over a period of weeks.

Self-help.   Don't remove a black toenail. Even if the toenail itself isn't firmly attached, it still protects the surface of the toe. If the toenail comes loose and falls off, put a small protective bandage over the end of the toe.

Professional help.   See a physician if there's acute bleeding under the nail and the pain is severe.

Painful or Black-and-Blue Toes

Causes and symptoms.   Stubbing your toe or hitting it against a hard object can produce a sprain or fracture. It may take up to 24 hours before you see any bruising.

Self-help.   Use rest, ice, and elevation to minimize swelling and further injury. Tape the injured toe to the adjacent normal toe to help keep it stable. Keeping weight off the foot is the most important part of initial treatment. Gradually resume activity in a day or two, after the pain has subsided.

Professional help.   When pain and disability persist for more than a week, consult a physician to make sure there isn't a more serious injury.

FOOT PAIN

Numbness in the Toes

Causes and symptoms.   Transient numbness and tingling are often felt in the feet during aerobic workouts that use stair climbing or step machines. Prolonged or repeated pressure on the small nerves in the front of the feet can interfere with sensation. Symptoms usually consist of numbness and tingling (but seldom pain) in the toes and the balls of both feet. However, discomfort may be felt anywhere in one or both feet. Symptoms are more likely to occur as the intensity and the duration of workouts increase. Numbness and tingling almost always go away within minutes after you stop.

Self-help.   Try changing your foot position by stepping more flat-footed. Loosening your shoes or wearing extra socks to cushion the feet may help.

Professional help.   When pain, tingling, or numbness persists, see an orthopedist or podiatrist to determine if there is an underlying bone or nerve problem. Individually fitted orthotic shoe inserts may be helpful.

Pain in the Top of the Foot

Causes and symptoms.   Tendons in the top of your foot, above the arch, can be irritated by friction and pressure if you wear tight shoes or tight ski boots. This is especially true for people who have high arches. Pain and tenderness are usually relieved when the source of pressure and irritation is removed.

Self-help. Protective pads and a change of shoes may quickly solve the problem. Try using two sets of laces—one for the top two or three pairs of eyelets, and the other set for the bottom pairs—so that you can adjust the fit and distribute the pressure on the top of the foot more comfortably.

Professional help. If pain persists, see an orthopedist or foot specialist to see if you have a stress fracture.

Pain in the Ball of the Foot (Metatarsalgia)

Causes and symptoms. Repeated impact causes strains and sometimes stress fractures—diffuse microscopic fractures of the front-foot (metatarsal) bones. Impact and swelling can also produce localized compression of nerves. Strains and stress fractures cause chronic pain that is felt in the ball of the foot (metatarsal arch) and within the foot itself. It's usually relieved by rest, but it can return once you resume impact activities. Nerve compression typically brings on burning or numbness between the third and fourth toes.

Self-help. Avoid high-impact activities (jogging, high-impact aerobics, and basketball) to allow the damage to heal. Insert soft arch pads and wear wider shoes. Gradually resume normal activities once the pain has subsided.

Professional help. If symptoms persist, see an orthopedist or podiatrist. Special imaging studies such as a bone scan, CT (computerized tomography) scan, or MRI (magnetic resonance image) may be needed to diagnose a stress fracture.

Pain in the Sole of the Foot (Plantar Fasciitis)

Causes and symptoms. Chronic impact can irritate the thick connecting tissues (plantar fasciae) that stretch over the sole of the foot. This irritation (plantar fasciitis) causes pain and tenderness anywhere on the bottom of the foot between the ball of the foot and the heel. The pain is aggravated by dancing and jogging, especially when done on hard surfaces.

Self-help. Change to shoes that provide more arch and heel support. Flexibility reduces the strain of repeated impact. Therefore, perform calf and heel stretches regularly (Figures 4.30 and 4.31).

Professional help. Persistent or recurring localized pain may respond to cortisone injections or prescription anti-inflammatory medications. Custom-designed shoe inserts (orthotics) help to re-distribute and dissipate impact forces.

Pain in the Bottom of the Heel

Causes and symptoms. Landing on a stone may bruise the base of the heel bone, causing localized pain with weight-bearing pressure on the heel. The repeated impact of jogging and aerobic dancing inflames the area and causes calcium deposits (bone spurs) to form at the front and underside of the heel bone. Impact may also irritate the bursa at the bottom of the heel. In either case, you may feel pain in front of the heel bone, on the bottom of the foot, during impact activities.

Self-help.   Avoid impact activities until the pain goes away. Wear shoes with thick, well-cushioned heels, and try placing a doughnut-type pad (sold in pharmacies) in the back of the shoe to keep pressure off sensitive areas.

Professional help.   Prescription anti-inflammatory drugs or cortisone injections provide relief for severe pain. You may need specially designed orthotics to reduce impact forces on the heel.

ANKLE INJURIES

Sprains and Fractures

Causes and symptoms.   Ankle sprains make up 30 to 50 percent of all sports-related injuries. Most often, sprains involve the outside part of the ankle where the ligaments stretch or tear as the foot turns underneath. Mild sprains are usually accompanied by low-grade pain and gradual swelling. Severe sprains cause immediate pain and rapid swelling. It's impossible to differentiate between a very severe sprain and a fracture without an X ray.

Self-help.   Apply ice to the sprained ankle as soon as possible. Keep the foot up, and support the ankle with either an elastic wrap or an elastic support. Avoid weight-bearing activities, but start ankle strengthening and rehabilitation exercises as soon as possible (Figures 8.1 and 4.33). Gradually resume normal activities once swelling has subsided.

Professional help.   Whenever there's immediate swelling and severe pain that prevents you from standing on your foot, X rays will help determine whether a fracture is present.

LOWER LEG INJURIES

Achilles Tendinitis

Causes and symptoms.   Inflammation of the Achilles tendon can occur after you increase your mileage, run over steep hills, or begin to work out on up-and-down terrain. It can also be the result of wearing new shoes that rub on the back of your heel. The tendon is tender to the touch. Discomfort can occur along the tendon anywhere between the back of the heel and the bottom of the calf. Usually, the heel and foot feel stiff, and you may notice a grinding sensation in the tendon when you simply move the foot up and down. Raising up the front of the foot or walking up and down stairs worsens the pain. Chronic inflammation weakens the Achilles tendon and increases the risk of a sudden rupture.

Self-help.   There's no quick fix for Achilles tendinitis. Cut down or stop the offending activity, apply ice, and try nonprescription medication such as ibuprofen. Putting heel lifts in the shoes may lessen the pain. Achilles stretching exercises are essential, and if you're not doing them already, start doing them before you resume activity (Figures 4.25, 4.30, and 4.31).

Professional help.   Serious tendinitis may require prescription anti-inflammatory medication, cortisone injections, or surgery.

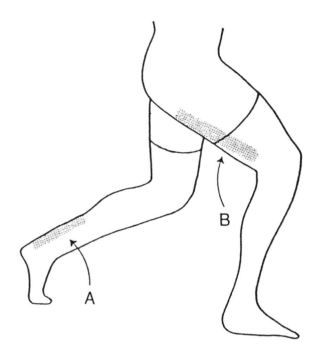

FIGURE 7.1 LEG INJURIES—LOCATION OF DISCOMFORT
A. Achilles tendinitis
B. Hamstring pull

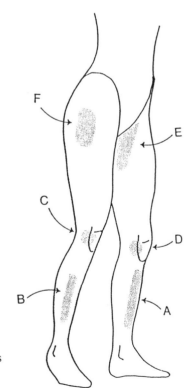

**FIGURE 7.2 LEG INJURIES—
LOCATION OF DISCOMFORT**
A. Shin splints
B. Anterior compartment syndrome
C. Iliotibial band tendinitis
D. Pes anserine tendinitis and bursitis
E. Groin pull
F. Hip (greater trochanteric) bursitis

Rupture of the Achilles Tendon

Causes and symptoms.   When you push off the front of your feet to run and jump, tremendous force is placed on the Achilles tendon. Lack of heel flexibility may increase the likelihood of rupturing the tendon. The pain is sudden and excruciating—like being shot in the heel. Walking is difficult and painful.

Self-help.   Apply ice, and see your doctor.

Professional help.   This injury requires immediate medical attention. You may need a cast to immobilize the foot and heel, or surgery to reattach the tendon. Recovery may take several months with a supervised rehabilitation program.

Rupture of the Calf Muscle ("Tennis Leg")

Causes and symptoms.   A quick jump or acceleration can tear the lower part of the calf muscle. This occurs so often among over-40 weekend tennis players that the injury is called "tennis leg." It feels as if you're suddenly hit in the back of the leg, and it hurts to stand on your toes. Some degree of swelling and bruising develops rapidly, and pain, stiffness, and tenderness persist for several days. Walking and stair climbing are painful, but symptoms usually resolve after several days.

Self-help.   Apply ice immediately. Use over-the-counter medications such as ibuprofen and acetaminophen, but avoid aspirin, which can aggravate the bruising and bleeding. Later, apply heat and do gentle calf-stretching exercises to aid recovery (Figures 4.25, 4.30, and 4.31).

Professional help.   If symptoms show no improvement within a week, see your doctor.

Calf Muscle Cramps

Causes and symptoms.   Muscle fatigue stems from repetitive overuse and occurs more often in warm weather. This may bring on disabling calf muscle cramps during long-distance running or after strenuous activity at racquet sports and basketball. The cramps usually involve both legs, and once they begin, even minor movements can trigger painful spasm.

Self-help.   Rest and fluid replacement will bring relief. Taking extra water before and during activity will help prevent calf cramps. Calf stretching before and after exercising can also help in the prevention of cramps.

Professional help.   Cramping that lasts for more than 24 hours should be evaluated by a physician.

Exercise-Related Phlebitis

Causes and symptoms.   Just being on your feet too long can irritate a varicose vein and cause a clot to form (superficial phlebitis). This condition may be uncomfortable, but the clot poses no risk of traveling. If you suffer a blow to the back of the leg or irritation from a nearby calf muscle rupture, a clot can form in a deep vein in the calf (deep thrombophlebitis). Usually, there's pain in the calf when you walk. Swelling in the foot and lower part of the leg indicates that the clot is blocking the vein and impeding drainage. With deep thrombophlebitis, a portion of the clot can break off and travel to the lung (pulmonary embolism). Symptoms of pulmonary embolism include shortness of breath, chest pain, and cough (sometimes, blood sputum as well).

Self-help. For superficial phlebitis, try nonprescription anti-inflammatory medication such as aspirin and ibuprofen. Wrap a warm towel around the affected part of the leg and then wrap a plastic bag over it to keep in the heat. Resume activity when you feel up to it.

Professional help. A superficial phlebitis can be felt as a firm, elongated, tender area and may require a prescription for anti-inflammatory medication. However, see a doctor for treatment if there's any indication at all of deep thrombophlebitis, such as calf pain and swelling.

Shin Splints

Causes and symptoms. Shin splints appear when you increase your running distance or after you play too much tennis or basketball on hard surfaces. Pain develops at the front of the shinbone (tibia). It's often worsened by weight-bearing activities, particularly downhill running.

Self-help. Switch to low-impact activities such as walking or swimming. Gradually resume normal activities when pain subsides. Avoid running on cement surfaces and playing tennis and basketball on hard courts.

Professional help. When symptoms don't disappear on their own, consult a physician to see if you are suffering from anterior compartment syndrome.

Anterior Compartment Syndrome

Causes and symptoms. The muscles along the outside of the shinbone, or tibia, raise the front of the feet. These muscles swell with blood and get almost 20 percent larger during vigorous running activities. They are wrapped in a nonelastic fibrous membrane that makes up the anterior compartment. If swelling is marked, pressure builds up in the anterior compartment and causes pain. Training or playing different sports on various surfaces (e.g., playing racquetball and then jogging on pavement) is a common cause. The pain typically occurs during exercise when you exceed a certain intensity or duration of activity.

Self-help. Pain usually disappears after several hours of rest. Ice and nonprescription anti-inflammatory medication help relieve the discomfort. Avoid jogging and other running activities until the pain diminishes. Gradually resume activity.

Professional help. If pain persists or if the symptoms become more intense, see a physician. In severe cases, surgery to open the anterior compartment may be necessary to relieve the pressure on the muscles.

KNEE INJURIES

Sprained Knee

Causes and symptoms. Falling while alpine skiing, sliding during baseball, and quickly changing direction playing football or basketball can all result in abrupt twisting, which can stretch and strain the ligaments inside the knee joint itself. With a severe sprain, the pain comes on immediately. If the sprain is mild, the knee may improve temporarily with resumption of activity, only to return after several hours of rest. Swelling in the knee occurs if there's any bleeding with the sprain.

Self-help.   Use RICE (page 113) and then gradually resume weight-bearing activities as symptoms subside. Anti-inflammatory medications such as acetaminophen or ibuprofen provide additional relief. Strengthening exercises for the quadriceps and hamstrings will help stabilize the knee joint (Figures 8.2, 8.3, 4.26, 4.27).

Professional help.   When the knee feels unstable, or when pain or swelling persist, see a physician. An MRI scan may be necessary to rule out a torn ligament or cartilage.

Torn Ligaments

Causes and symptoms.   The same activities that cause sprains can result in torn ligaments if the twisting and pulling forces are great enough. Some people feel or hear a "pop" with a complete tear of the ligament. Ligament tears cause almost immediate pain and swelling of the knee, indicating bleeding inside the joint.

Self-help.   RICE treatment (page 113) minimizes the swelling until you can get professional help.

Professional help.   Anytime the knee joint feels wobbly, is unstable, or pain prevents you from bearing weight, obtain medical attention immediately.

Torn Cartilage

Causes and symptoms.   Sudden twisting or changing direction while running can cause the cartilage (meniscus) that lines the knee to rupture or split. Pain usually comes on suddenly and tends to develop either on the inside (medial) or outside (lateral) part of the knee. Fluid can build up in the joint, and weight bearing rapidly becomes painful. Sometimes the cartilage is torn simply because of continued wear and tear; symptoms will come on gradually or for no apparent reason. With any torn cartilage, pain characteristically worsens when you walk upstairs, but you may not feel much pain going down. Squatting is painful, but kneeling usually doesn't cause pain. Nevertheless, it hurts to get up and down. Sitting is comfortable (even with the legs crossed), and jumping straight up and down is usually not a problem. Occasionally, pieces of cartilage separate, giving the sensation of something loose inside the joint. This may impede movement and actually cause the joint to lock so you can't straighten it.

Self-help.   Use RICE (page 113) and anti-inflammatory drugs such as ibuprofen. Avoid aspirin, which may aggravate bleeding around the injured area. Most partial tears heal as long as you limit your weight-bearing activities.

Professional help.   If pain or swelling persists or recurs, see an orthopedic specialist. You may need MRI or other special imaging studies to make the diagnosis. When healing doesn't occur naturally, surgical removal through a scope (arthroscopy) may be necessary.

Swelling of the Knee

Causes and symptoms. The repeated impact of running and jumping can irritate the synovial membranes that line the knee joint. Synovial tissue normally manufactures fluid that lubricates the knee joint, and when it's irritated or inflamed for any reason, it produces more fluid. People who already have arthritic knees are most likely to experience knee swelling after exercise.

Self-help. Ice, rest, and ibuprofen or acetaminophen provide relief. Choose lower-impact activities, try to play on softer surfaces (clay instead of concrete tennis courts), and wear shoes with good shock-absorbing soles.

Professional help. If the pain in the swollen knee is severe, if the swelling occurs immediately after trauma or a fall, or if you find it difficult to move your knee, see a physician. If the swelling doesn't decrease within 24 hours, the fluid can be removed using a syringe and needle. The swelling may be caused by bleeding from ligament or cartilage damage, or by the presence of irritating crystalline material (gout or pseudogout). Examining the joint fluid usually pinpoints the specific cause.

Tendinitis on the Outer Side of the Knee

Causes and symptoms. Pain may result from overuse of the tendon that stretches between the bone above the hip and the outside of the knee. This tendon is known as the *iliotibial band*. Usually, there's tenderness over the bone on the outside of the knee, and there may be pain, grating, and stiffness at the start of exercise. Sometimes the symptoms go away during activity but return after you finish. The knee joint itself isn't swollen, and it's able to maintain its normal range of motion.

Self-help. Ice and anti-inflammatory drugs such as ibuprofen are helpful. It's important to temporarily stop the activity that causes the irritation. You may want to start cross-training so that you can cut down on the intensity and duration of the irritating activity. Exercises to stretch the iliotibial band are the key to long-term treatment (Figure 4.23).

Professional help. Most irritation to the iliotibial band responds to self-help. If pain persists, you may need a cortisone injection and a professionally supervised rehabilitation program. Additional evaluation can rule out a hip problem as the source of the pain.

Tendinitis and Bursitis at the Inner Side of the Knee
(Pes Anserine Bursitis and Tendinitis)

Causes and symptoms. Pain and tenderness over the bone at the inside (medial) lower part of the knee can be caused by running, swimming the breaststroke, climbing, and stepping, all of which irritate the tendon and bursa at that site (pes anserine tendinitis and bursitis). As with other tendinitis at the knee, the joint itself is unaffected and free of swelling. At the start of exercise, there may be grating and stiffness that go away during activity but return at rest.

Self-help. Ice and ibuprofen are helpful. Cut down or stop the activity causing the inflammation. Stretching and strengthening the thigh muscles (quadriceps and hamstrings) are the most important aspect of long-term treatment (Figures 8.2, 8.3, 4.26, and 4.27).

Professional help.   Most often, tendinitis and bursitis respond to self-help treatment. But if pain persists, seek professional evaluation. Cortisone injections or prescription anti-inflammatory medication and a professionally supervised rehabilitation program may be needed.

Tendinitis at the Top and Front of the Knee

Causes and symptoms.   In kneecap (patellar) and thigh muscle (quadriceps) tendinitis, tenderness and pain are felt at the top of the kneecap where tendons of the quadriceps muscle attach. The knee joint itself isn't affected, but there may be grating and stiffness felt at the top surface of the knee at the start of exercise. This tends to go away during activity and to return later at rest. Usually, pain worsens going downhill or down steps, and prolonged sitting (especially with the legs crossed) is uncomfortable. People with kneecap tendinitis find it difficult to get up and down into a squatting position, but once they are down there, they feel more comfortable.

Self-help.   Use ice and anti-inflammatory medications, and cut down or stop the activity causing the inflammation. Stretching and strengthening the quadriceps muscles prevent long-term problems (Figures 8.2, 4.26, and 4.27).

Professional help.   Most often, kneecap and thigh muscle tendinitis clear up with self-help treatment. If pain persists, have a professional evaluation for further treatment and a supervised rehabilitation program.

"Water on the Knees" (Prepatellar Bursitis)

Causes and symptoms.   A direct blow to the kneecap, the repeated pressure of kneeling, or the continued strain during alpine skiing may cause fluid buildup under the kneecap (patella). Other than the pain that arises from a direct blow or fall, the fluid accumulation is painless.

Self-help.   The fluid is gradually reabsorbed over one to two weeks. Usually, the condition improves on its own as long as there's no further irritation.

Professional help.   If there's severe or persistent pain associated with the swelling, consult with a physician for X rays to determine whether there's a fracture of the kneecap.

Kneecap Inflammation (Chondromalacia Patella)

Causes and symptoms.   Repeated rubbing between the underside of the kneecap and the surface of the underlying bone during running activities may gradually cause an inflammation known as chondromalacia patella. People with this condition feel stiffness and pain in the front part of the knee before they run. Wearing worn-out shoes and running on irregular or slanted surfaces may aggravate the condition. The stiffness lessens after a few minutes of running, but it returns within 30 minutes of stopping, often lasting into the night. Kneeling, going down steps, and running downhill are particularly painful.

Self-help.   Anti-inflammatory medications such as aspirin (it's okay in this case because there's no bleeding) and ibuprofen relieve some of the discomfort. But the most important step is to decrease the distance you run or to stop running altogether for a period of time. New athletic shoes and running on flat terrain may help.

Professional help.   Professional help is rarely needed.

THIGH AND HIP INJURIES

Muscle Spasms and Cramps

Causes and symptoms.   The large muscles in the front of the thighs (quadriceps) are particularly vulnerable to fatigue and cramping when long-distance biking, running, or hiking depletes body fluid levels. Spasms may be disabling and be triggered by even the slightest movement.

Self-help.   Fluids, ice packs, and rest correct the problem.

Professional help.   When wooziness or light-headedness doesn't go away or if dehydration is severe, medical help with intravenous fluid and salt may be needed.

Delayed Muscle Soreness

Causes and symptoms.   The weekend or occasional exerciser whose muscles are not well trained will feel soreness 12 to 24 hours after vigorous or sustained activity.

Self-help.   Nonprescription anti-inflammatory medications help control discomfort, but the soreness subsides after several days of rest. Gradually increase activity to build up strength and endurance.

Professional help.   If soreness continues for more than two or three days, you may have a more serious injury. See your physician.

Groin Pull

Causes and symptoms.   The upper inner thigh muscles can be pulled or strained with sudden starts, stops, jumps, and lateral movements. Older athletes who don't maintain their leg flexibility and strength are at the greatest risk. Pain and spasm are sudden and often disabling.

Self-help.   For the first 24 to 48 hours, use RICE measures (page 113). After 24 to 48 hours, try heat and ibuprofen or aspirin. Gentle flexibility exercises can help to restore function (Figure 4.22). Once pain has diminished, strengthening the inner thigh muscles helps to prevent further problems (Figure 4.28).

Professional help.   Severe pain associated with swelling and bruising may indicate a serious muscle tear. If this is the case, see your doctor. If you have persistent groin pain while bearing weight, see your physician to determine if you have a hip or pelvic fracture.

Thigh Bruise ("Charley Horse")

Causes and symptoms.   With a mild bruise, pain and stiffness often don't occur until five to ten minutes after activity. With more severe injuries, pain and stiffness come on quickly. You may notice swelling from bleeding in the muscle (hematoma).

Self-help.   Use the RICE treatment (page 113), and wait at least 48 hours before you gradually resume activities. You may use ibuprofen or acetaminophen, but stay away from aspirin, which may aggravate any bleeding. Heat is helpful after 48 hours.

Professional help. Sometimes the injured muscle turns into a tender and painful lump several weeks after the injury. If there's any pain or loss of function, consult with your physician.

Bursitis of the Hip (Greater Trochanteric Bursitis)

Causes and symptoms. The bursa at the side of the hip (greater trochanter of the femur) is a common site of irritation. The bursa is tender when you press on it, and some people are unable to sleep on that side.

Self-help. Use an anti-inflammatory drug such as ibuprofen. Do stretching exercises to increase flexibility (Figure 4.23).

Professional help. If the pain doesn't improve, a cortisone injection into the inflamed bursa can provide relief.

Hip, Leg, and Pelvic Fractures

Causes and symptoms. Any bone that's even mildly weakened, or osteoporotic, is more likely to break with a fall. If there's a severe fracture of the hip (actually the upper part of the leg bone), almost immediately it's impossible to bear weight or even move without excruciating pain. With incomplete fractures, there may be only moderate pain when you walk. Stress fractures of the thighbone (femur) are rare but are sometimes experienced by thin women who are long-distance runners.

Self-help. Self-help is not appropriate.

Professional help. Persistent groin, hip, mid-leg, pelvic, or otherwise unexplained knee pain after a fall shouldn't be ignored. Most hip fractures require surgery to prevent further damage and to restore good function. Although surgery isn't appropriate for a fractured pelvis, there should be a professionally supervised rehabilitation program. When standard X rays are not effective, a bone scan, MRI scan, or CT scan may be necessary to make an accurate diagnosis.

Aseptic Necrosis of the Hip

Causes and symptoms. Occasionally, a fall damages the blood supply to the top of the leg bone, causing the death (necrosis) of the ball of the hip joint. When there's persistent hip or groin pain despite normal-appearing X rays, aseptic necrosis is a possibility.

Self-help. Self-help is not appropriate.

Professional help. An MRI or CT scan may be needed. A supervised rehabilitation program is mandatory. In severe cases, artificial hip replacement may be required.

BACK INJURIES

Muscle Strains and Pulls

Causes and symptoms. Twists, pulls, and improper lifting techniques are the most common triggering events for acute strains on either side of the spine. But the major underlying causes of back muscle strains and pulls are insufficient flexibility and strength. Abnormal side-to-side curvature of the spine (scoliosis) also creates a structural imbalance, increasing the likelihood of activity-related strains and spasms. Spasms in the lower back (lumbar) muscles and strains of the upper (thoracic) muscles are also common. Often the pain is so severe that it's nearly impossible to straighten up and turn.

Self-help. For painful strains, use RICE measures (page 113) for the first 24 hours. After the first 24 hours of a severe strain, or if the pain is not severe, heat and anti-inflammatory medication such as aspirin or ibuprofen can be used. Once the pain diminishes, strengthening and flexibility exercises are the cornerstone of rehabilitation and prevention (Figures 4.3, 4.4, 4.10, 4.17–4.19, and 4.21).

Professional help. If the pain and spasm are severe, you may need prescription pain relievers or muscle relaxants. When symptoms are incapacitating, worsen, or persist for longer than a week, consult with your physician.

Tailbone (Coccyx) Pain

Causes and symptoms. The coccyx can be bruised or even fractured after falling on your tailbone or with repeated bumping and bouncing on a hard seat. Sitting is very uncomfortable, and tenderness lasts for a week or more.

Self-help. You can lessen discomfort by taking acetaminophen or ibuprofen and sitting on an inflatable doughnut or pillow, which takes the pressure off the injured area.

Professional help. Other than prescription pain relievers, additional treatment is rarely needed.

Slipped (Herniated) Disk

Causes and symptoms. The strains of heavy weight training or pushing can produce a bulging (herniation) of one of the disks between the vertebrae in the lower (lumbar) spine. A herniated lumbar disk may also come on more gradually with repeated stress on the lower back from jogging or rowing. Initially, pain is felt in the lower back, but the area is usually not tender to the touch. The pain may be felt in the buttocks on one side or down the back of the leg, and it's generally worse when you cough or sneeze. People are usually more comfortable lying on their sides with the knees bent; sitting and bending tend to aggravate the pain.

Self-help. Bed rest and ibuprofen or acetaminophen allow the bulging disk to shrink. Afterward, a stretching and strengthening program for the back is important (Figures 4.8–4.10 and 4.20). Substitute swimming for activities such as jogging and rowing.

Professional help. Prescription pain relievers are often needed. If you have persistent pain or if you develop numbness or weakness in the foot or leg, see your doctor for additional diagnostic studies and treatment.

Collapsed Vertebra (Compression Fracture)

Causes and symptoms.   Repeated impact from jogging or aerobic dance, or the strain of lifting, may bring on a collapse (compression fracture) of an osteoporotic vertebra. Localized aching and pain develop rapidly in the spine at the site of the fracture, usually in the mid or lower back. The pain usually disappears within one or two weeks, but it may linger with severe fractures.

Self-help.   Rest and ibuprofen or acetaminophen are the cornerstones of treatment. Once you feel better, start a walking program, but avoid impact activities.

Professional help.   X rays are necessary to confirm the diagnosis and to rule out the possibility of an underlying problem such as a tumor, which might have also weakened the bone. Prescription pain relievers are often necessary.

Sciatica

Causes and symptoms.   The major causes of sciatica are irritation of the lower lumbar nerve roots from a bulging disk and pressure on the sciatic nerve by bone spurs or tight buttock muscles. A weak back and a lack of flexibility can bring it on. Sciatica is characterized by severe pains starting in one buttock and going down the back or side of the leg, often all the way to the foot. There may also be accompanying lower-back pain. While the symptoms are usually felt only on one side, nerve root compression caused by the bone spurs of an arthritic spine (spinal stenosis) may cause problems on both sides. If the cause is a herniated disk, you may feel better lying down but feel worse sitting or bent forward. If the source of sciatic irritation is lumbar spinal stenosis, then you will be more comfortable sitting or bent forward.

Self-help.   Acetaminophen, aspirin, or ibuprofen is usually not enough to control the pain. Rest and non-weight-bearing activities usually control the problem. Once you're feeling better, hip and lower-back flexibility and conditioning exercises are essential to help prevent recurrence (Figures 4.8–4.10, 4.20, and 4.25). However, you should proceed with professional guidance and supervision in order to resume activity safely and avoid further injury.

Professional help.   Prescription analgesics are usually needed to control the pain. When symptoms don't improve within several days, further medical evaluation is necessary to determine the precise diagnosis and the most appropriate treatment.

ABDOMINAL INJURIES

Abdominal Muscle Pull or Strain

Causes and symptoms.   Sudden abdominal pains may come on after twisting, pulling, or receiving a direct blow or kick to the abdomen. Delayed abdominal muscle pains may result from doing too many sit-ups, leg raises, or stomach crunches. Aching is usually steady, and when you press on the abdomen, it hurts more when you tighten the muscles than when you let them relax. The aching may last days or even weeks.

Self-help.   Heat, acetaminophen, and rest usually correct the problem.

Professional help.   If the abdomen becomes swollen, tender, and black-and-blue, check with your physician to see if there is serious bleeding within the abdominal muscles. If pain persists, see your doctor to find out if there are other causes.

Hernia

Causes and symptoms.   Increased pressure within the abdomen, often caused by heavy lifting or straining, can cause vulnerable tissues in the groin, abdominal wall, or navel to bulge, stretch, or tear. An underlying weakness may be present because of prior surgery or injury. Very often hernias are painless, but if adjacent tissues get twisted or caught up in the hernia sac (*incarcerated* hernia), there is steady pain. The weakened tissues don't heal themselves, and a hernia either remains stable or enlarges over time.

Self-help.   Avoid heavy lifting and straining.

Professional help.   For a hernia in the groin area, see your physician regarding possible surgical repair. Localized pain, cramps, and nausea could represent a loop of intestine caught up in the hernia. This requires emergency attention.

GENITAL INJURIES

Testicular Trauma

Causes and symptoms.   A direct kick or blow, and even the impact from bouncing on a bicycle seat, can bruise unprotected testicles.

Self-help.   Rest and support are generally all that's needed. Don't take aspirin, which could aggravate any bleeding inside the testicles or scrotal sac.

Professional help.   If there's severe pain or persistent swelling, see a urologist.

Penile Numbness

Causes and symptoms.   A long bicycle ride on a narrow or improperly adjusted seat can put direct pressure on the pudendal nerve at the base of the penis.

Self-help.   The numbness will diminish after several hours and needs no special treatment. You can prevent it by using a wide and fully padded bicycle seat.

Professional help.   Professional evaluation is seldom needed.

Vaginal Trauma

Causes and symptoms.   Vaginal bruises and tears occasionally occur with bicycle accidents or in water skiing after you fall while being towed.

Self-help.   Avoid aspirin, which could aggravate bleeding. Use acetaminophen or ibuprofen for pain. Rubber pants for water skiers will provide protection.

Professional help.   If there's bleeding, significant swelling, or difficulty with urination, see your physician right away.

CHEST INJURIES

Muscle Stitch

Causes and symptoms.   Intense aerobic activity may bring on sudden sharp pain in the upper abdomen, anywhere in the chest, and occasionally in the shoulders. These muscle spasms generally occur within the first 10 to 15 minutes of activity and make breathing difficult. The pain from a muscle stitch can be quite intense, but it subsides rapidly when you slow down or stop activity.

Self-help.   Warming up and accelerating more slowly will prevent muscle stitches.

Professional help.   When chest discomfort persists in spite of stopping, or if it recurs predictably, see your doctor without delay. You could have a heart- or lung-related problem.

Chest Wall Strain

Causes and symptoms.   The muscles in the breast area (pectorals) are subject to delayed muscle soreness after intense weight training and rowing, or after direct blows. Other common sites of irritation and tenderness are along the sides of the breastbone (sternum), where cartilage connects the ribs and sternum. The chest wall can be identified as the site of the discomfort because you can reproduce the pain by squeezing the pectoral muscles or by pressing along the sides of the sternum.

Self-help.   Chest wall strains usually improve on their own within a few days. Heat, aspirin, acetaminophen, or ibuprofen provide substantial additional relief.

Professional help.   Pain in the chest is an alarming symptom. If there's any associated shortness of breath or any question about the origin of the pain, see your physician immediately.

Breast Trauma

Causes and symptoms.   Direct impact during martial arts or racquet sports may bruise the breasts. Breast tissue is very sensitive, and contusions are very painful.

Self-help.   The initial use of ice and possibly compression with an elastic chest binder helps to minimize the swelling. Avoid aspirin and instead use acetaminophen or ibuprofen for pain. Chest protectors should be used when doing martial arts.

Professional help.   Breast contusions subside within several weeks, and professional help is seldom necessary.

Rib Fractures

Causes and symptoms. Osteoporosis increases the likelihood of rib fractures. The pain is severe and sharp, and it feels worse when you twist, turn, breathe, or cough. You may even feel a grinding or moving sensation when you breathe, and the area over the fracture is almost always tender to the touch.

Self-help. The symptoms diminish significantly within one to two weeks but often linger if you remain active. Use nonprescription pain medication other than aspirin. Binding the chest with an elastic bandage or rib belt (sold in pharmacies or medical supply stores), or splinting the area by lying against a pillow, can sometimes restrict movement enough to reduce the pain.

Professional help. Without an X ray, there's no way to tell whether or not a rib is fractured, and even then a mild fracture may not be identified. If you experience a severe or sudden increase in shortness of breath, or if there's a clear bulge in the rib, see your doctor. If you have any prior history of breast or prostate cancer, X rays are important to rule out any possibility of cancer involvement in the ribs.

Fractured Collarbone (Clavicle)

Causes and symptoms. Falls during cycling or jogging are the most common causes of clavicle fractures. There is a bulge over the middle or outer part of the collarbone (clavicle), and pain comes on immediately. The pain is worse when you raise your arm but better when you bend your elbow and hold the arm against your chest.

Self-help. Use ice and keep your arm and hand immobilized against your chest. Take acetaminophen or ibuprofen for pain, but avoid aspirin, which may aggravate bleeding.

Professional help. See your doctor for X rays and for a fitted sling or harness to keep the clavicle stable. Healing typically takes four to six weeks, and surgery is rarely needed. After healing has occurred, a supervised rehabilitation program is needed to restore strength and mobility at the shoulder.

NECK AND SHOULDER INJURIES

Neck Strains

Causes and symptoms. Most exercise-associated pain in the upper back or neck (trapezius muscle) results either from muscle strain or from the aggravation of underlying arthritis in the neck (cervical spine). Neck strains tend to linger because we use these muscles to support the head and arms during sedentary activities such as typing, writing, talking on the phone, and driving.

Self-help. Rest, heat, and nonprescription analgesics are helpful. The primary long-term treatment is a flexibility program for the neck and shoulders (Figures 4.1, 4.2, and 4.11–4.13).

Professional help. Sharp or shooting pain that travels to the neck and arm may indicate nerve pressure from bone spurs in the neck. Another possible cause is a disk in the neck (cervical disk). This requires further evaluation, including X rays.

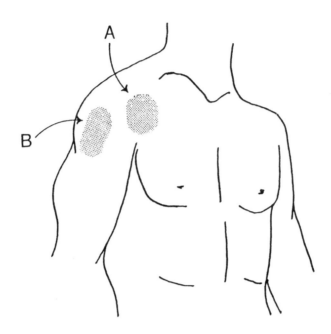

FIGURE 7.3 SHOULDER INJURIES—LOCATION OF DISCOMFORT
A. Rotator cuff strain
B. Shoulder bursitis

Shoulder Rotator Cuff Tendinitis

Causes and symptoms. The tendons of the rotator cuff, located in the front of the shoulder above the armpit, can suffer overuse strains. Pain is often worse when you reach behind you. Pain comes on when you hold your arms out straight away from your side, or when you bend your elbow 90 degrees and turn your arm at the shoulder so that your forearm and hand are pointing straight down, perpendicular to the ground. You can feel the pain of rotator cuff tendinitis during activity. Often the pain is worse at night, interrupting sleep.

Self-help. Stop the activity, apply ice, and take over-the-counter anti-inflammatory medications. Do shoulder exercises to maintain flexibility and strengthen the rotator cuff (Figures 8.5–8.8).

Professional help. When self-help is not enough, see your physician to find out if you have a rotator cuff tear. Prescription anti-inflammatory medications or cortisone injections can provide significant relief.

Shoulder Rotator Cuff Tears

Causes and symptoms. The same activities that bring on rotator cuff tendinitis can cause a rotator cuff tear. Tears may come on abruptly with rapid, forceful movements, or they may occur gradually with overuse. The symptoms of a gradual rotator cuff tear are the same as for rotator cuff tendinitis. A sudden tear may cause disabling pain.

Self-help. Self-help measures are the same as those for rotator cuff tendinitis.

Professional help. When pain is severe, and when it persists or worsens, you need professional attention. You may need an MRI scan to make the diagnosis or you may need an arthrogram, a special X ray in which a dye is injected into the shoulder joint. Leakage of this dye out of the joint indicates a rotator cuff tear. If there's a significant tear, a supervised rehabilitation program is essential. Sometimes surgery is the only way to repair a torn rotator cuff.

Adhesive Capsulitis

Causes and symptoms. If you don't maintain shoulder flexibility when the shoulder is injured or inflamed, the capsule of the shoulder joint can scar and shrink. This comes on gradually over weeks or months. The reduction in mobility may be so severe that you can't raise your arm higher than the shoulder.

Self-help. Shoulder flexibility exercises are essential (Figures 4.2, 4.13, 8.5, and 8.6). It's easier to do them under a hot shower or while using a heating pad over the shoulder.

Professional help. In severe cases, the only way to restore mobility is to break down the adhesions by moving the shoulder. This is done under anesthesia.

Shoulder Bursitis

Causes and symptoms. Overuse from swimming (freestyle, backstroke, and butterfly), tennis (serving), and weight training (lifting overhead) can inflame the major bursae of the side of the shoulder. The shoulder aches, and it hurts to press on the area above the bursae. Discomfort can worsen while resting after activity, and it can keep you up at night. When you raise your arm straight out at your side, the shoulder begins to hurt as the arm becomes horizontal and then again when it's overhead and nearly vertical.

Self-help. Rest, ice, and nonprescription anti-inflammatory medications provide relief.

Professional help. Prescription anti-inflammatory medications or cortisone injections into the inflamed bursae provide additional relief.

Shoulder Sprain, Separation, and Dislocation

Causes and symptoms. Falling on your hand so that your arm is stretched behind you can tear one or more of the ligaments that attach the end of the collarbone (clavicle) to the head of the shoulder. The injury is classified as either a sprain, a mild separation, or a severe separation, depending on the severity of the tear and how many of the ligaments are affected. With sprains and mild separations, pain and stiffness gradually build. With severe separations, the degree of pain and instability is much greater, and it comes on immediately.

Self-help. Apply ice and immobilize your shoulder by bending your elbow 90 degrees and holding the arm in against your chest. Acetaminophen and ibuprofen help control the pain. Avoid aspirin because it increases the likelihood of bleeding.

Professional help. If the end of the clavicle bulges out, if pain is severe, or if it's very difficult to move the shoulder, get immediate medical help.

ARM AND ELBOW INJURIES

Triceps Strain and Tendinitis

Causes and symptoms. Using ski poles, doing too many push-ups, or lifting too much weight can bring on either overuse irritations or acute strains of the triceps muscle and tendon. Pain is felt in the back of the arm near the elbow, and it's worse when you try to straighten the bent arm against resistance.

Self-help. Usually, rest, ice, and over-the-counter anti-inflammatory medications provide relief. Once the pain has subsided, do triceps stretching (Figures 4.2, 4.11, and 4.13) and strengthening exercises (Figures 4.5–4.7 and 4.15).

Professional help. Professional help is rarely necessary.

Biceps Muscle Tear or Rupture

Causes and symptoms. If excessive force is placed on the muscle, part of the biceps in the upper arm can rupture. This typically occurs while you're doing arm curls or pull-ups on an overhead bar. Pain is usually felt close to the shoulder (the end of the biceps that usually ruptures), and a distinct bulge or lump forms in the middle of the upper arm as the torn muscle recoils. The area may become black-and-blue after 24 to 48 hours.

Self-help. Ice and acetaminophen or ibuprofen will control the pain. Avoid aspirin, which could aggravate bleeding. Once the pain and swelling decrease, work on strengthening with weights or resistance machines.

Professional help. Ordinarily, the muscle is not reattached surgically because there is enough remaining muscle to do most activities. See a sports medicine or orthopedic physician if there's any question.

Tendinitis at the Outside of the Elbow (Tennis Elbow)

Causes and symptoms. Overuse irritation where the forearm muscles attach to the outside of the elbow is commonly known as tennis elbow. It can also occur with other racquet sports, golf, bowling, bicycling, and martial arts. Poor backhand form, weak forearm muscles, stiff or highly strung racquets, and a grip that's too narrow will all contribute to the strain at the tendon attachment. The pain generally occurs during the activity. Pain and tenderness may be so severe that simply lifting a briefcase or turning a doorknob is excruciating.

Self-help. Ice and nonprescription anti-inflammatory medications help relieve the pain. Stay away from the activity long enough to allow the inflammation to subside, then start a forearm-strengthening program (Figures 4.14 and 8.10–8.12). An elastic forearm strap (found at a pro shop or sporting goods store) can reduce the pull of the muscle on the elbow. It may help to change to a larger grip or to an oversize racquet that is strung at a lower tension. Improving backhand technique or changing to a two-handed backhand may prevent a recurrence.

Professional help. Cortisone injections and prescription anti-inflammatory medications control severe pain. But they do not substitute for rest and a subsequent forearm-strengthening program.

Tendinitis at the Inside of the Elbow (Golfer's Elbow)

Causes and symptoms. A condition similar to tennis elbow occurs at the inside of the elbow. It afflicts golfers who hit the ground too often or who use stiff clubs. It can also affect tennis and squash players who use excessive forehand topspin.

Self-help. Self-help measures are similar to those for tennis elbow.

Professional help. Prescription anti-inflammatory drugs and cortisone injections control severe pain. However, they don't substitute for rest and a subsequent forearm-strengthening program (Figures 4.14 and 8.10–8.12).

Bursitis of the Elbow

Causes and symptoms. Bumping the point of the elbow can bring on swelling in the bursa overlying the bone. Swelling due to fluid collection can reach golf-ball size. The swelling is usually painless except for the bump on the bone itself.

Self-help. Swelling generally resolves after seven days, but it can last for a month or more. In the meantime, avoid leaning on the elbow.

Professional help. Ordinarily the fluid doesn't need to be removed. If the swollen area becomes reddened, warm, or tender, see your doctor. There may be an infection that requires antibiotics and drainage of the fluid.

WRIST AND HAND INJURIES

Sprained Wrist

Causes and symptoms. Excessively bending the wrist—usually by falling on your hand—can sprain ligaments. Any part of the wrist may be affected. The most common cause is falling on an outstretched palm and bending the hand back, known as hyperextension. Hyperextension sprains usually affect the thumb side of the under part of the wrist. Landing on the outside of the hand and bending it under causes a sprain on the underside of the wrist opposite the thumb. With either type of sprain, almost any movement is painful.

Self-help.   Use RICE measures (page 113). A splint or brace (sold in medical supply stores and many pharmacies) to immobilize the wrist might be helpful. Acetaminophen and ibuprofen provide additional pain relief. Gradually resume activity when pain and swelling have diminished.

Professional help.   If pain and swelling are severe, fail to improve within 24 hours, or return as you resume activity, you must get an X ray to determine if you have a fracture of the forearm bones (radius and ulna) or the wrist (carpal) bones themselves. Persistent pain in the wrist may indicate a fracture in one of the wrist bones. This may not heal without professional attention. If a fracture isn't treated, it could lead to permanent arthritis and loss of wrist function.

Tendinitis of the Wrist

Causes and symptoms.   Paddling and rowing may produce overuse irritation of the tendons on the back of the wrist. Gripping dropped handlebars during long bicycle rides can irritate the tendons on the thumb side of the wrist. The quick chops and slices of squash and racquetball may inflame the tendons on the side of the wrist. Pain is brought on during the activities themselves.

Self-help.   Take nonprescription anti-inflammatory medications, and cut back on or avoid the activities that cause the inflammation.

Professional help.   Professional medical help other than prescription anti-inflammatory medication is rarely needed.

Ganglion Cyst

Causes and symptoms.   Weaknesses sometimes arise in the sleeve of a tendon or in the capsule of one of the joint spaces in the wrist. A pea-size firm, smooth lump (ganglion cyst) can appear. It's usually painless, and it doesn't ordinarily affect the function of the wrist.

Self-help.   A ganglion cyst is harmless but rarely goes away on its own.

Professional help.   If the cyst is bothersome, it can be surgically removed by an orthopedist. The thick fluid within the cyst can be removed with a syringe, but it is almost certain to recur.

Carpal Tunnel Syndrome

Causes and symptoms.   The nerve that provides sensation to the thumb, the second finger, and part or all of the middle finger passes through the wrist (carpal) bones. This passageway through the wrist (carpal tunnel) may already be narrowed by arthritis. Bowling, weight training, skiing, racquet sports, rowing, and cycling (gripping dropped handlebars) can produce additional wrist irritation and swelling, which pinch the nerve. Symptoms include numbness and tingling in the thumb and first two fingers, as well as pain and aching in the wrist, forearm, or elbow that occurs at night. People often wake up and shake their hand to relieve the discomfort.

Self-help.   Stop the activity, and take an anti-inflammatory drug such as ibuprofen.

Professional help. If symptoms persist, cortisone injections may help. Wearing a splint in bed to keep the wrist straight and the hand slightly back may prevent nighttime pain. If pain or numbness is severe and doesn't improve, surgery may be needed to take the pressure off the nerve.

Ulnar Nerve Compression

Causes and symptoms. At the outside of the wrist, the nerve may be compressed or pinched as it passes through the fleshy portion of the outside of the palm. Racquet sports, weight lifting, alpine skiing, golf, and martial arts may cause the pressure on the nerve—either because of the strain from a tight grip or from direct trauma. Symptoms include tingling and numbness in the fourth and fifth fingers, possibly associated with aching in the outside part of the palm. There may be pain behind the inside part of the elbow ("funny bone"), primarily at night.

Self-help. Discontinue the offending activity. Nonprescription anti-inflammatory medications often help.

Professional help. If symptoms don't disappear, surgery may be needed to take pressure off the nerve.

Tendinitis of the Hand

Causes and symptoms. Gripping an oar or bicycle handlebars for long periods of time may inflame the tendons in the palm of the hand. Hand movements may become stiff and painful, and you may feel a sudden "trigger" sensation when opening or closing the fingers.

Self-help. In addition to RICE measures (page 113), proper cushioning and padding in the palm are essential. Place a piece of foam padding inside a light cotton glove. Also, extra foam padding for handlebars can be found at most bicycle shops.

Professional help. Surgery to relieve the pressure on the ulnar nerve is rarely needed.

Sprained Thumb (Skier's Thumb)

Causes and symptoms. Sprains of the ligament that attach to the inside part of the thumb are the most common of all ski injuries. They occur when a skier attempts to break a fall with the outstretched hand while holding a ski pole. There is pain and swelling primarily on the inside part of the base of the thumb. Pinch strength is usually diminished.

Self-help. Use RICE measures (page 113), and if the sprain is mild, immobilize the thumb with a hand splint (sold in medical supply stores and many drugstores).

Professional help. If there's any instability or loss of strength in the thumb, you may need a cast to immobilize the thumb for four to six weeks. This should be followed by a supervised rehabilitation program. Severe injuries may require surgical repair, which if delayed may result in permanent disability.

Sprained Finger

Causes and symptoms. Fingers can be sprained when they're bent back suddenly. The impact and pulling produce swelling and stiffness around the joints at the end or middle of the finger.

Self-help. RICE measures (page 113) are usually enough. A finger splint (sold in medical supply stores or pharmacies) should be worn at night and during the daytime to prevent further irritation. Once the swelling and pain lessen enough to restore comfortable movement, you can gradually resume activities that use the hand.

Professional help. For severe pain and swelling, especially if there's any bruising at or near the injured joint, get an X ray of the finger and hand. These symptoms suggest that there could be a fracture, either in a wrist bone (often below the thumb) or in one of the fingers. If a wrist bone fracture isn't properly identified, it may not heal correctly, resulting in permanent arthritis.

Dislocated Finger

Causes and symptoms. Occasionally, a sudden blow knocks a finger bone out of joint so that you're unable to bend it. It will be stiff and possibly swollen, and pain may or may not be pronounced.

Self-help. It is risky to try to put a dislocated finger back into place yourself.

Professional help. You should see a physician (your regular doctor, an orthopedic physician, or an emergency room physician) or a sports medicine professional to put the finger back into place. You may need an X ray to rule out the presence of a fracture.

FACE AND HEAD INJURIES

Nosebleeds and Nasal Injuries

Causes and symptoms. Nosebleeds may follow a direct blow to the face. They may also occur spontaneously after spending several days in dry air—skiing, hiking, or climbing at high altitudes. Spontaneous nosebleeds are painless.

Self-help. Apply direct pressure by squeezing with your thumb over the side that's bleeding. Put ice against the bleeding side until you're sure the bleeding has stopped.

Professional help. If bleeding recurs or if it continues to drain down the back of the throat, the nose needs to be packed. If a blow to the nose has caused swelling and pain, X rays will determine if there has been a nasal fracture.

Corneal Abrasions and Irritations of the Eyes

Causes and symptoms. Mild injuries to the surface of the eye (cornea) produce a scratchy feeling in the eye. More serious injuries can bring on acute pain, sensitivity to light, and blurred vision. Uncomplicated corneal abrasions heal themselves in 24 hours.

Self-help. Never rub the eye. Always wear goggles or eye protection while cycling, skiing, swimming, and playing indoor racquet sports.

Professional help. If there's any continued irritation, bleeding, visual impairment, light sensitivity, or persistent pain, medical attention is mandatory. Persistent scratchiness in the eye may indicate the presence of a foreign body or a more serious abrasion.

Middle-Ear and Sinus Problems

Causes and symptoms. The effects of any congestion in the eustachian tube and sinus cavities are worsened by sudden changes in barometric pressure associated with scuba diving and the rapid descent of downhill skiing. Symptoms include diminished hearing as well as pain and pressure in the ears, cheekbones, and above the eyes. For divers, pressure buildup can be severe enough to bring on a rupture of the eardrum, causing pain and a sudden loss of hearing. Most ruptured eardrums heal on their own. Hearing usually returns within one or two weeks.

Self-help. Decongestant medications such as pseudoephedrine (*Sudafed*) and phenylpropanolamine (*Entex*) can expand blocked sinus and eustachian tube openings.

Professional help. If congestion or loss of hearing persists, see a physician. If you have a history of heart or blood pressure problems, check with your doctor before using decongestant pills.

Concussion and Loss of Consciousness

Causes and symptoms. A blow to the head may stun or knock you out. You may be dazed and experience headache or temporary loss of memory.

Self-help. Apply ice to any swelling on the scalp. If there's no loss of consciousness, return to activity if you feel up to it.

Professional help. If you have any loss of consciousness, severe headache, or persistent confusion, you need to be evaluated immediately. You should be observed closely for any change in alertness and response. Any persistence of symptoms or change in behavior in the days or week following a head injury could indicate bleeding under the skull (subdural hematoma). These symptoms mandate further evaluation and possibly a CT scan or MRI scan of the head.

THERMAL INJURIES

Prickly Heat

Causes and symptoms. Sweat glands may become irritated with exercise in hot, humid weather. Red, itchy blisters and bumps break out at the sweat pores.

Self-help. Wear well-ventilated clothing. Keep the affected area clean and dry. The irritation will subside on its own. For some people, antiperspirants can be irritating with prickly heat.

Professional help. If the area around the rash becomes red and swollen, medical evaluation is advised.

Heat Cramps

Causes and symptoms. Vigorous activity in hot or humid weather causes sweating, resulting in severe body fluid depletion. Muscles active during exercise begin to cramp, and the cramps tend to wander from muscle to muscle. People who take diuretic medications are more susceptible.

Self-help. Rest and replace fluids with diluted juice or water.

Professional help. Professional help may be needed if symptoms do not improve.

Heat Exhaustion and Heatstroke

Causes and symptoms. Prolonged exercise in either hot or humid weather can produce over-heating and dehydration. The symptoms of heat exhaustion include nausea, irritability, headache, dizziness, and goose bumps on the skin. Confusion, vomiting, diarrhea, and possibly coma and convulsions signify heatstroke. Sweating may or may not accompany these symptoms.

Self-help. Stop what you are doing. Find a cool place, lie down, and replace lost body fluids with water or diluted fruit juice (any commercial electrolyte-replacement solution will do). "Tanking up" with fluids before you start on a hot day will give you a reserve to prevent heat exhaustion.

Professional help. Severe heat exhaustion, especially if there are painful muscle cramps, responds more quickly to intravenous fluids. The symptoms of heatstroke require immediate emergency medical assistance.

Sunburn

Causes and symptoms. The two factors that influence the development of sunburn are the amount of sun exposure (how much and how long) and the pigmentation of the skin. In lightly pigmented people, the ultraviolet-B radiation of sunlight rapidly brings on redness, which reaches maximal intensity about 24 hours after exposure. Sunlight is reflected by snow and water, amplifying the ultraviolet radiation. Severe sunburns are actually second-degree burns with blistering and subsequent peeling of the skin. Other symptoms may include fever, chills, and nausea.

Self-help. Anti-inflammatory medication such as aspirin or ibuprofen reduces the symptoms. Cool soaks may provide comfort as well. Wear sunscreens, a hat, or a visor, and engage in outdoor activities early or late in the day, if possible. Ultraviolet-B intensity at those times is only one-tenth of what it is at the height of the day.

Professional help. If blisters, nausea, weakness, and lethargy persist, see your doctor.

Frostbite

Causes and symptoms. Damage to the skin from freezing primarily affects the hands, feet, ears, and nose. The risk of cold injuries is increased by windy conditions, wet clothing, alcohol or tobacco use, and high altitudes. Superficial frostbite appears as flat, white patches associated with the decreased sensation of the involved skin. The numbness lasts for only a few days. As it rewarms, the skin swells, blisters, becomes mottled, and turns bluish purple before it returns to normal. Deep frostbite represents more serious freezing damage that may extend all the way to the bone. With deep frostbite, the skin remains cool and mottled even after rewarming. Over a period of three to six weeks, the damaged tissue shrivels and dies.

Self-help. Rewarm the involved part of the body in cool or slightly warm water, but don't rewarm deep frostbite injuries until you're sure that there will be no additional cold exposure. The most extensive skin damage occurs when thawed tissues become frozen again.

Professional help. After the initial thawing has taken place, follow up with a physician who will monitor healing. Dead tissue may have to be removed surgically.

BITES AND STINGS

Insect Bites

Causes and symptoms. Bee, hornet, wasp, and fire ant venoms cause swelling, itching, and burning, usually confined to the site of the bite. The extent of the reaction depends on the number of bites.

Self-help. Remove any insect parts, and cover the bite with a mixture of meat tenderizer and rubbing alcohol or a paste of water and baking soda. Over-the-counter cortisone creams reduce the itching, and oral antihistamines may be helpful for more extensive reactions.

Professional help. Light-headedness, difficulty breathing, or a raised, itching rash (hives) in a part of the body away from the bite signify a general allergic response to the venom. Subsequent stings can bring on a more serious and life-threatening reaction called anaphylactic shock. Consult your physician or an allergy specialist about a prescription insect sting kit and the advisability of desensitization shots.

Aquatic Bites and Stings

Causes and symptoms. Many jellyfish, sea urchins, stingrays, and varieties of coral protect themselves with potent toxins that cause burning, itching, and painful rashes at the site of contact. Rarely, life-threatening allergic reactions occur in susceptible individuals.

Self-help. Cover the area of contact with a mixture of meat tenderizer and rubbing alcohol, or bathe the area in vinegar. This inactivates the venom and relieves the burning and itching. If you have a puncture wound from a stingray, soak the area in very hot water to help inactivate the toxin.

Professional help. If you develop wheezing, generalized hives, itching on the palms, or a thickened tongue, see your physician.

Poison Ivy and Contact Dermatitis

Causes and symptoms. Between 50 and 85 percent of the U.S. population are allergic to the resins and oils in plants such as poison ivy, poison oak, and poison sumac. Depending on the degree of sensitivity, these people may develop itching, blistering, scaling, and crusting within six hours to several days after contact. Most of the skin damage has been done by the time the reaction appears.

Self-help. If you've had contact with a plant to which you know you are sensitive, wash your skin (including under the fingernails) and your clothing as soon as possible. Apply cortisone creams and calamine lotion. Sedating antihistamines such as diphenhydramine (*Benadryl*) and chlorpheniramine (*Chlortrimeton*) are helpful at night. (If you have prostate problems or glaucoma, check with your doctor first.)

Professional help. For severe or generalized reactions, cortisone medication given by pill or injection is much more effective than topical medications.

Hives

Causes and symptoms. Hives (urticaria) may be brought on by allergic reactions, and in rare instances, exercise itself can trigger them. In some people, rapid rises in body temperature during aerobic exercise release the chemical histamine, which causes urticaria. The rash is raised, smooth, and very itchy. It appears on any part of the body, and usually on both sides equally.

Self-help. Nonprescription antihistamines are helpful in most cases.

Professional help. Exercise-induced hives can cause seriously low blood pressure and even collapse. If you have hives and feel that it's related to activity itself (not an allergy or bite), consult your physician.

EXERCISE-RELATED INFECTIONS

Boils and Impetigo

Causes and symptoms. Staphylococcal and streptococcal bacteria are present on the skin. The irritation of the buttocks experienced by rowers and riders can cause localized infections (boils) often involving the hair follicles. The same bacteria can spread and cause red, crusting, itching-surface infections that are usually located in body folds.

Self-help. Apply warm compresses to boils to promote drainage and healing. Try nonprescription antibiotic ointments for small areas of impetigo.

Professional help. Large boils should be drained. Severe or widespread infections require oral antibiotics.

Herpes Simplex (Fever Blisters)

Causes and symptoms.   Many people harbor herpes simplex virus in the skin of the mouth and lips. Exposure to sunlight can trigger a blistering, unsightly, contagious, and sometimes painful rash on or near the lip. Typically, this recurring rash erupts during the first days at the beach, on the water, or in the mountains.

Self-help.   Keep the rash clean and dry. Protect the area from additional sun exposure by applying zinc oxide.

Professional help.   Prescription acyclovir (*Zovirax*) ointment may speed healing. When flare-ups occur predictably, taking acyclovir capsules for several days prior to anticipated sun exposure prevents most acute episodes.

Fungal Infections

Causes and symptoms.   Fungi called dermatophytes thrive in the warm, moist areas between the toes, in the groin, and sometimes under the arms. Dermatophytes cause athlete's foot and jock itch. In the inner thighs, the groin, and under the arms, the rash is flat, red, and sharply bordered. The rawness and cracking between and under the toes can be painful and incapacitating.

Self-help.   Wear cotton socks, well-ventilated clothing, and comfortable shoes. Keep the involved areas as dry as possible. Try over-the-counter creams and powders containing tolnaftate, undecyclenic acid, and miconazole.

Professional help.   Infections that don't respond to nonprescription remedies may require stronger topical or oral medication, which is available only by prescription.

Lyme Disease

Causes and symptoms.   Lyme disease is a bacterial infection transmitted by infected ticks. Ticks are found primarily in the Northeast from Massachusetts to Virginia; in the Midwest, mainly in Minnesota and Wisconsin; and occasionally in the West. They attach themselves to warm-blooded animals (including humans) who brush against them in the grass, bushes, and low vegetation of the woodlands where they live. The ticks are about the size of a pencil dot and feed from May through August. To infect someone, the ticks must feed for about 24 hours. This leaves ample time to search and remove them after possible exposure. The earliest sign of infection is a flat, red rash with a "bull's-eye" center and a diameter of typically two inches or more. The rash slowly expands in a circle from the site of the bite, and then goes away without treatment after days or weeks. Fever, joint aches and swelling, muscle aches, and persistent fatigue may follow.

Self-help.   If you're exercising in a tick-infested area, wear long sleeves and tuck your pants into your socks. If you are outside in a high-risk area, survey your entire body for ticks after you come inside. Light-colored clothing provides a better background for spotting any ticks you pick up.

Professional help.   If you think you may have been exposed to Lyme disease or if you have any of the symptoms described above, check with your doctor regarding blood tests and appropriate antibiotics.

8

GETTING BACK INTO ACTION

Injuries tend to take a greater toll on you as you age. Your tendons, ligaments, and joints, which may already be somewhat stiff, are even less supple when you're injured. Rehabilitation means restoring you to your normal state of health. If you're physically active, a rehabilitation program will help you regain at least the level of function and conditioning you had achieved before you were injured.

Effective rehabilitation helps to prevent the permanent loss of flexibility, strength, and exercise capability that often follows an injury. The goals of a personally tailored rehabilitation program to overcome injury are straightforward. They include

- preserving or restoring flexibility in the injured or unused part of the body
- rebuilding strength as soon as possible without causing additional tissue damage
- maintaining a level of aerobic fitness without compromising healing or making the injury worse
- getting back to an exercise regime that will make future injuries less likely

Rehabilitation is an *active* process. For the person over 40, it's crucial to start a rehab program as soon as you're able. Although you may have the guidance and support of sports medicine professionals, the responsibility for performing the exercises to regain your strength and function belongs to you.

ANKLE AND FOOT INJURIES

Ankle Sprains

Anytime you have a severe sprain, a rehabilitation flexibility, strengthening, and activity program should take place under the guidance and supervision of a sports medicine professional. Even for those sprains with only modest swelling and pain, returning to activity too soon may increase the likelihood of reinjury.

Rehab at home. An important part of rehabilitation and prevention of reinjury is to maintain and increase your Achilles tendon flexibility. After your pain has subsided, do the back-of-the-thigh (hamstring) stretch (Figure 4.25) and calf and heel stretches (Figures 4.30 and 4.31) at least three times a week. Also try the two following exercises.

1. *Walk on your toes and heels.* Walk on your toes and heels to strengthen the muscles that stabilize the ankle joint. Stand on your toes and then your heels for 20 to 30 seconds while you hold on to a table or chair for support. Do this daily.
2. *Towel curl.* See Figure 8.1. Do this exercise daily during rehab.

Exercise tips and precautions. To maintain aerobic fitness while you're healing, try cycling, swimming, or running in deep water wearing a flotation jacket. As you get back on your feet, start with casual then brisk walking on level terrain. Be patient, and if problems recur, check with your physician or sports medicine professional.

Heel Injuries (Achilles Tendinitis and Bursitis of the Heel)

Heel injuries interfere with running and jumping. Serious injuries require specific, professionally supervised rehabilitation exercises.

Rehab at home. Concentrate on increasing your Achilles tendon flexibility. Back-of-the-thigh

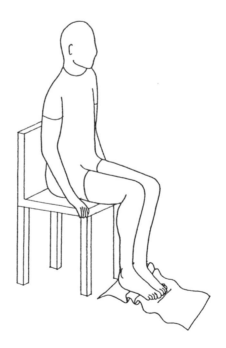

FIGURE 8.1 TOWEL CURL Put a towel on a smooth floor and sit on a chair with your feet flat. Using your toes, bunch or curl the towel up under your foot. Keep your feet *flat* on the floor at all times. Do this daily during rehab.

stretches (Figure 4.25) along with calf and heel stretches (Figures 4.30 and 4.31) strengthen the Achilles tendon and prevent further injury. Do them at least three times a week.

Exercise tips and precautions. The best way to overcome mild or moderate recurring discomfort in the back of the heel is to cut down on running. Maintain your fitness by doing activities that don't require you to push off on your toes. Rowing and swimming are excellent aerobic alternatives.

LEG, HIP, AND THIGH INJURIES

Shin Splints

It's essential to stop the activity that's causing your shin splints, and it may take several weeks before the pain subsides.

Rehab at home. Do exercises for the Achilles tendon (Figures 4.25, 4.30, and 4.31) at least three times a week.

Exercise tips and precautions. Once the pain is gone, start activity slowly at about two-thirds of your normal intensity. Then increase your effort gradually over four to eight weeks. Exercise on softer surfaces. Play tennis on clay-type courts, run on surfaces other than concrete, and do aerobics on a thicker mat. Also, wear well-cushioned shoes, even when you're not exercising. Walking on hard pavement in leather-soled shoes can prolong the problem. If pain returns immediately when you resume exercise, consult your physician.

Knee Injuries

Before you start working to rehabilitate the knee, it's essential to have a professional evaluation.

Rehab at home. Rehabilitation must include stretching exercises for the muscles and tendons in the front and back of the thigh (quadriceps and hamstrings). (See figures 4.24 and 4.25.) Do the quadriceps exercises at least three times a week. Lunges (Figure 4.26) and minisquats (Figure 4.27) require no special equipment. You can do additional strengthening exercises with three- to five-pound ankle weights (sold in any sporting goods store):

1. *Knee extensions.* See Figure 8.2.
2. *Leg curls.* See Figure 8.3.

More vigorous strengthening can be done under a therapist's supervision using resistance machines.

Exercise tips and precautions. As with all overuse injuries, the key ingredient in rehab is time. For serious knee injuries, plan on giving the injured knee up to six weeks of rest before you resume the particular activity (usually involving running or jumping) that caused the problem. The amount of time that you need for healing will vary, and you should check with an exercise professional for advice on when to resume activity if there is any question in your mind. Until the pain and tenderness have subsided, other activities such as swimming, rowing, skating, and cross-country skiing provide good aerobic alternatives. Avoid stair-climbing machines and cycle cautiously, if at all.

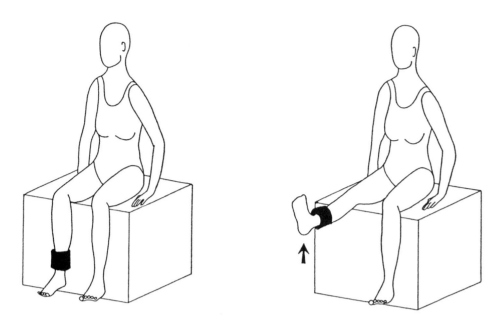

FIGURES 8.2a, 8.2b **KNEE EXTENSIONS** Sit on a chair or bench with your feet hanging down. (Ankle weights, which are sold in any sporting goods store, are optional.) Slowly raise your right foot until your knee is almost straight. Hold for a slow count to 10. Then slowly lower your foot to the starting position. Repeat 10 times. Take a deep breath and relax. Do the same exercise with the left leg.

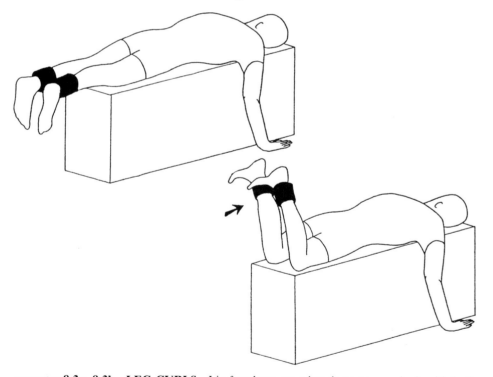

FIGURES 8.3a, 8.3b **LEG CURLS** Lie facedown on a bench or on your bed, with both legs straight. (Ankle weights, which are sold in any sporting goods store, are optional.) Slowly raise your feet until the knees are at a 90-degree angle. Pause for no more than one or two seconds and slowly lower your feet until the legs are straight. Keep your back flat so that your hips are in contact with the bench. Repeat 15 to 20 times.

Hip Pain (Bursitis)

Bursitis over the side of the hip is a common overuse irritation experienced by runners.

Rehab at home.   The key to effective rehabilitation is increasing the flexibility in the side of the leg from the outer pelvis to the knee (iliotibial band). Stretching the iliotibial band will reduce the friction over the bursa during running or climbing. A beneficial exercise is the outer-hip (iliotibial band) stretch (Figure 4.23). It should be done three times a week.

Exercise tips and precautions.   For hip pain that's caused by a direct blow to the side of the hip or the result of overuse, work on upper-body exercises until you can move the leg comfortably. Gradually resume your regular activity as the pain diminishes. If discomfort persists or returns, consult with your sports medicine professional.

Groin Pull

Strains in the inner upper thigh muscles may be very slow to heal. The key elements for effective rehabilitation include stretching, strengthening, gradual resumption of activity, and time.

Rehab at home.   Maintaining the full range of motion at the hip is very important, and these exercises should be done at least three times a week. The best way to do this is to apply heat while you stretch. Once the pain has lessened, do the groin stretch (Figure 4.22) while applying heat to the upper thigh. Place a hot towel around the upper thigh, and then wrap a large plastic garbage bag over it to keep the heat in.
    For strengthening the inner muscles of the thighs, try thigh squeezes (Figure 4.28).

Exercise tips and precautions.   You may need to allow several weeks for the pain to subside. It may be difficult to maintain an alternative aerobic program until you feel more comfortable. Work on your upper body, and consult with a sports medicine professional if you're not improving.

Hamstring Pull

Pulls and strains in the muscles in the upper back of the thighs (hamstrings) occur more often in the over-40 exerciser. Weekend tennis, racquetball, and squash players who haven't maintained their hamstring muscle flexibility are at the greatest risk.

Rehab at home.   Once rest and ice have lessened the acute pain, start a gentle stretching program. Do the hamstring stretch (Figure 8.4) at least three times a week.

Exercise tips and precautions.   Gradually resume activity—first walking, then walk-jogging. Be patient, because a hamstring strain may take several weeks to heal fully. If you're not making progress or if problems recur, a sports medicine professional can provide further guidance for rehabilitation.

BACK INJURIES

Lower Back Strains and Sprains

Lower back strains and sprains are among the most disabling exercise-associated injuries in people over 40.

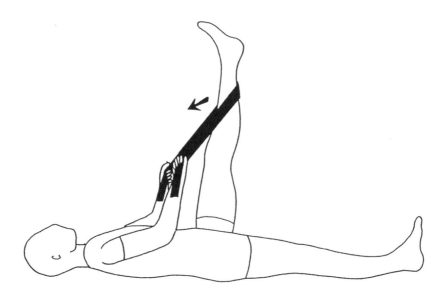

FIGURE 8.4 HAMSTRING STRETCH You may do this exercise by pulling a rope or towel that is looped around the calf, or by having a partner gently raise the leg for you. Lie flat on your back and keep the affected leg straight at all times. Slowly raise this leg toward your head until you begin to feel tightness. Continue to breathe normally; don't hold your breath. Hold for 30 seconds and then let the leg down. Applying heat by wrapping a hot towel around the painful area also helps during stretching.

Rehab at home.   Once pain is under control, there are two basic elements in a back rehabilitation program. First, you need to strengthen the abdominal muscles and the muscles that control the pelvis. Second, you need to improve the flexibility in the lower back, hamstring muscles, outer hip (iliotibial bands), and Achilles tendon. The following exercises will help prevent further injury. Perform them at least three times a week.

> Lower-back and buttock stretch (Figure 4.8)
> Pelvic tilt (Figure 4.10)
> Complete body stretch (Figure 4.16)
> Mid-back stretches (Figures 4.17 and 4.18)
> Outer-hip (iliotibial band) stretch (Figure 4.23)
> Front-thigh (quadriceps) stretch (Figure 4.24)
> Back-of-the-thigh (hamstring) stretch (Figure 4.25)
> Calf and heel stretch (Figure 4.30)

Exercise tips and precautions.   Absolute rest is rarely necessary for treating back strains. It's important for you to work on maintaining your aerobic and general muscular fitness. The best way to accomplish this is by swimming or cycling. Avoid jogging, because of the impact; stay away from racquet sports because of the twisting involved; and omit the weight-training exercises, which may strain the lower back. Rowing machines can pose problems because of the additional load on the mid and lower back. Sometimes it takes six to eight weeks for back strains to heal fully. If pains worsen or if you're not getting better, additional medical evaluation is advisable.

NECK INJURIES

After you reach the age of 55 or 60, arthritic changes in the neck (cervical spine) are the rule rather than the exception. You may not even feel any discomfort, since very often bone spurs visible on an X ray are not accompanied by pain. Even without pain, the arthritic cervical spine will be less flexible.

Neck and Shoulder Strains

When a strain is present, it's difficult to keep the supporting muscles of the neck relaxed. When you raise your arms straight out in front or push your jaw or head forward, the muscles in your neck and upper shoulder must pull back at the same time.

Rehab at home.   Heat, pain relief, and careful attention to posture are the most important factors in the early rehabilitation of neck and shoulder strains. Once the pain and irritation subside, strengthen the neck muscles with pushing exercises. Do the following at least three times a week:

Head and hand push. Take either palm and press it against your forehead. Push your head against your palm. Push back with your palm with an equal amount of force so that your head doesn't move. Hold for a slow count to 10. Relax. Repeat the exercise on the right side of the head with your right palm against your head, over the ear. Follow with the left side. For the back of your head, clasp your fingers and place both palms against the back of the head and follow the same pattern. Relax. Do this twice in the morning and twice at night.

Other exercises you can do at home are the neck, shoulder, and arm stretch (Figure 4.2), the shoulder shrug (Figure 4.12), and the outer-shoulder (triceps) stretch (Figure 4.13).

Exercise tips and precautions.   For aerobic fitness, walk or jog with your head and shoulders as relaxed as possible. Try swimming the backstroke or the crawl. Avoid activities where your head is bent back, such as swimming the breaststroke or cycling with low handlebars. Relax your neck and shoulder muscles by sitting up straight and close to your desk or the steering wheel in your car. Keep your shoulders back when you stand, and don't carry heavy briefcases, purses, or shoulder bags.

SHOULDER, ARM, AND WRIST INJURIES

Shoulder Injuries

Your shoulder has the greatest freedom of movement of any joint in your body. This broad range of motion is possible only because the shoulder relies mainly on muscles and tendons (instead of rigid ligaments) for its stability.

Rehab at home.   The most important part of any shoulder rehabilitation is to move the arm comfortably through as full a range of motion as possible. Do these easy exercises at least three times a week.

Making circles with your arms (Figure 8.5).
Walking up the wall with your hand (Figure 8.6)

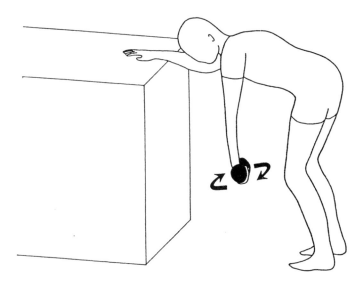

FIGURE 8.5 MAKING CIRCLES WITH YOUR ARMS Hold on to the back of a stationary object with one hand. With the other hand, hold a one- or two-pound weight (or a 16-ounce can), bend your knees, lean forward, and let your arm hang straight down. Keeping your elbow straight, make small circles with your arm (clockwise or counterclockwise, it doesn't matter). First make the circles a few inches in diameter and enlarge them until the circles are about two feet around. Make them slowly. And if you feel pain, cut back.

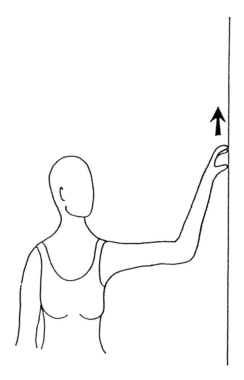

FIGURE 8.6 WALKING UP THE WALL WITH YOUR HAND Stand with the line of your shoulders perpendicular to the wall. Start at the side of your chest and walk your fingers slowly straight up the wall until your hand is above your head and your elbow is almost straight. Repeat five times, twice daily.

Exercise tips and precautions. You can maintain your overall aerobic fitness during the rehabilitation period by walking, jogging, or cycling.

To prevent rotator cuff and further shoulder injury, do the following exercises at least three days a week:

>   Arm pushes (Figure 8.7)
>   Inward arm rotation (Figure 8.8)
>   Outward arm rotation (Figure 8.9)

If the shoulder strain is severe or if pain doesn't subside after several days of rest, professional evaluation and guidance are strongly advised.

Elbow Strains and Tendinitis

Most people feel the discomfort of tennis or golfer's elbow in the outside or inside part of the elbow for months before they seek treatment. The first step in rehabilitation is to let the inflammation diminish. The only way to accomplish this is to stop the activity, at least temporarily.

Rehab at home. Once the pain in the elbow lessens, you're ready to start a stretching and strengthening program for the wrist and forearm. Repeat the following at least three times per week:

Hand stretch. Hold the affected arm out straight. Use the other hand to gradually bend the affected wrist back, and hold for a count of 10. Then, still keeping the arm straight, bend the wrist down for a count of 10. Repeat this sequence four times.

Wrist curls and reverse wrist curls (Figure 4.14).

Squeeze the ball. Squeeze a soft rubber ball or tennis ball for three seconds and then relax. Repeat this 10 to 20 times with both hands. Do this twice a day.

Wrist bend—forward (Figure 8.10).

Wrist bend—back (Figure 8.11).

Wrist turnover (Figure 8.12).

If any one of these exercises is painful, see a sports medicine professional for further guidance.

Exercise tips and precautions. During rehab, maintain your fitness by walking, jogging, or doing aerobic dance. Avoid rowing and other exercises that use the arm. When the pain at the elbow affects your daily activities or if the pain doesn't diminish with rest, see a physician to discuss additional treatment.

Wrist Sprains

Anytime you have a severe sprain, a rehabilitation flexibility, strengthening, and activity program should take place under the guidance of a sports medicine professional. Even for those sprains that produce only modest swelling and pain, returning to activity too soon may increase the likelihood of reinjury. A severely swollen or painful wrist should always be X-rayed. An inadequately healed wrist may lead to arthritis or long-term disability.

Rehab at home. Once the pain and swelling have subsided, start the same kind of gentle stretching and strengthening exercises described in the section on the elbow.

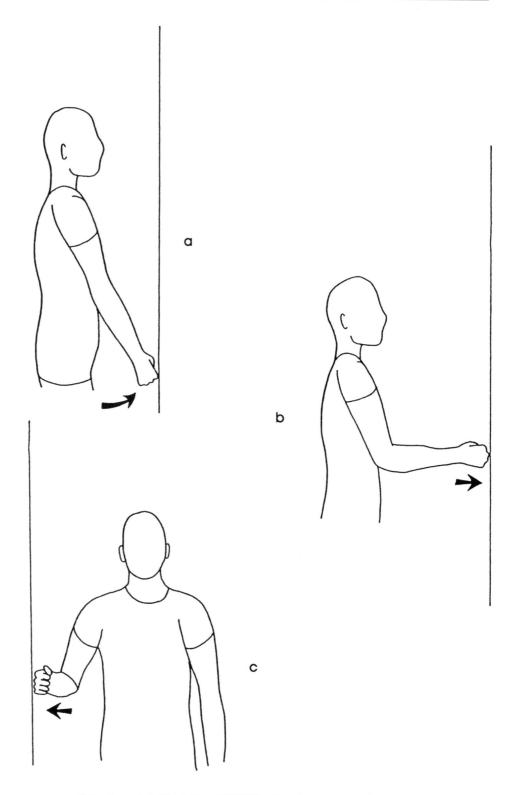

FIGURES **8.7a through 8.7f   ARM PUSHES**   Stand one to two feet away from the wall. Push against the wall with your hand and hold each position for a slow count to 10. Relax your neck and breathe slowly. Pause before you change to the next position. Repeat the sequence at least twice daily.

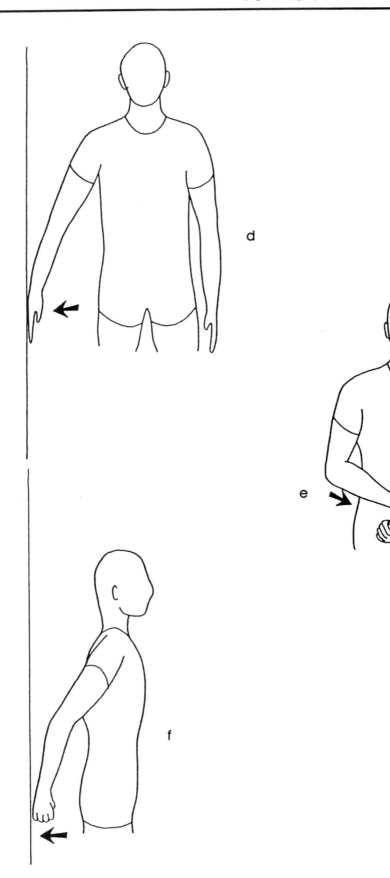

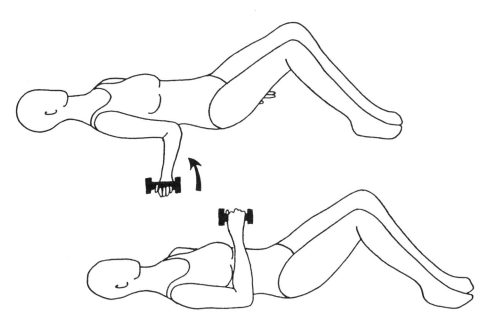

FIGURES 8.8a, 8.8b   INWARD ARM ROTATION   Lie on your back with your head comfortably supported. Hold a two- or three-pound weight (sold in any sporting goods store). Start with your arm against your chest, your forearm flat against the floor, and your elbow bent 90 degrees. Keeping the elbow against your chest, slowly rotate the arm until the forearm is in a vertical position. Slowly rotate the arm back to the starting position and repeat 10 times. Relax. Switch to the other side, and do the same routine.

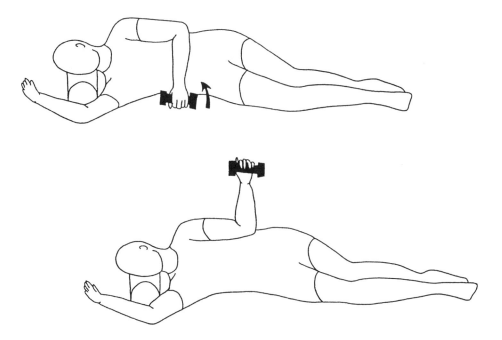

FIGURES 8.9a, 8.9b   OUTWARD ARM ROTATION   Lie on your side. Hold a two- or three-pound weight. Start with your arm against your chest and your elbow bent 90 degrees. Keeping the elbow against your chest, slowly rotate the arm to raise the hand up and out. Slowly let down the arm and repeat 10 times. Relax. Switch to the other side and do the same routine.

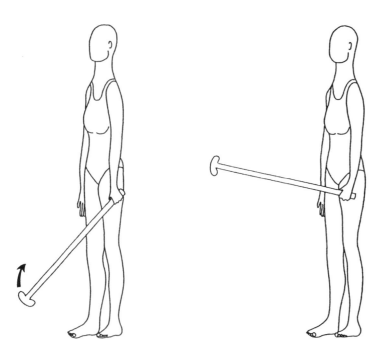

FIGURES **8.10a, 8.10b   WRIST BEND—FORWARD**   Hold a golf club in your hand. Keeping your arm straight and using only your wrist, raise the club to the front. Slowly let the club down. Repeat 10 times. Then repeat with the other hand.

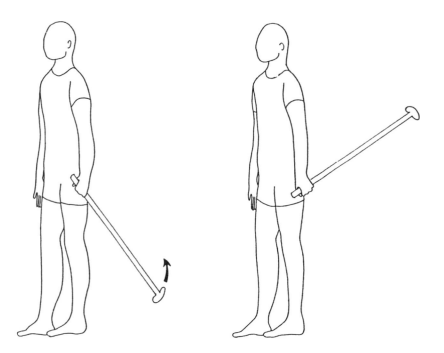

FIGURES **8.11a, 8.11b   WRIST BEND—BACK**   Hold a golf club. Keeping your arm straight and using only your wrist, slowly raise the club in back of you. Slowly bring it back to the starting position. Repeat 10 times. Then repeat with the other hand.

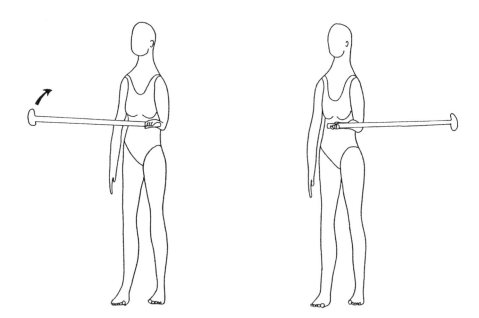

FIGURES 8.12a, 8.12b   WRIST TURNOVER   Hold a golf club straight across and in front of your body with your palm facing down. Keeping your elbow bent at 90 degrees, and using only your wrist, slowly bring the club up and over to the outside. Slowly reverse the movement to bring the club back to the starting point. Repeat 10 times. Then repeat with the other hand.

Exercise tips and precautions.   As with elbow and forearm rehab, walk, jog, or do aerobic dance, none of which requires the use of your hands. If you experience repeated or increased discomfort with these exercises, seek the guidance of a sports medicine professional.

EXPERT HELP AND WHERE TO FIND IT

Sports medicine takes in many medical areas, and it involves a variety of professionals. The professionals most likely to play a role are physicians, physical therapists, podiatrists, nurses, and exercise physiologists. Depending on the licensure laws in your state, these people may function independently or under the direct supervision of a physician.

Each of these professionals has a unique role to play in the treatment and rehabilitation of your exercise-related problem. It can be confusing, since almost any of them can be called a "sports medicine specialist."

Your local hospital may have a sports medicine clinic or referral service for treatment and rehabilitation of activity-related injuries. Check with club pros and coaches, trainers, and fitness instructors, as well as exercise partners and other sports medicine consumers, for their advice. Be both aware and well informed about the quality of the programs available to you.

Physicians

Orthopedic surgeons, emergency room doctors, family practitioners, internists and physiatrists (physical medicine and rehabilitation specialists) are the physicians who typically handle adult sports medicine problems. These physicians have graduated from either an allopathic (M.D.

degree) or osteopathic (D.O. degree) medical school. Although there are a growing number of multidisciplinary postgraduate training programs in sports medicine, until recently there was not even a sports medicine certification examination offered by the American Board of Medical Specialties (the primary organization overseeing certification in 23 medical and surgical specialties).

In 1993 the boards of Family Practice, Pediatrics, Emergency Medicine, and Internal Medicine joined to write a fellowship curriculum and examination leading to a Certificate of Added Qualifications in Sports Medicine. Professional expertise is also provided by orthopedic surgeons or physical medicine and rehabilitation specialists. There are several independent organizations that offer examinations and certificates of competence in sports medicine. However, none has the same stature and recognition as the American Board of Medical Specialties.

Podiatrists

Podiatrists are independent, licensed medical professionals whose practice is limited to problems involving the feet and ankles. After completing college-level preprofessional education, they have obtained a degree from an accredited school of podiatric medicine. In many locales, podiatrists work in concert with orthopedic surgeons in handling activity-related foot, knee, and leg injuries. As is the case with other medical professionals, their expertise and scope of responsibility vary with the extent of their training. Some podiatrists have completed postgraduate in-hospital surgical training programs and are qualified to perform foot surgery in hospitals. Podiatrists are skilled in treating overuse injuries due to running and jumping; they also provide treatment when there are underlying arthritic problems with the feet.

Chiropractors

Chiropractors are independent, licensed practitioners who have obtained a degree from a school of chiropractic medicine. Much of their practice centers on the treatment of back problems caused by strains, sprains, and spinal misalignment. In addition to massage and manipulation, chiropractors use many of the same therapeutic modalities (such as heat and ultrasound) used by physical therapists.

Physical Therapists

Physical therapists complete a college curriculum before taking a comprehensive certification examination. They are licensed by the state in which they practice. Physical therapists provide rehabilitation services that are prescribed by a physician, although they usually have broad discretion in how they fill that prescription. In many states, physical therapists are permitted to act independently within the scope of their training and expertise. Nevertheless, insurance coverage and reimbursement often require the initial evaluation and oversight of a licensed medical or osteopathic physician.

Nurses

Licensed registered nurses are most likely to be involved with cardiac rehabilitation programs. Specially trained cardiac nurses may administer and monitor exercise sessions for high-risk people who are recovering from a heart attack or heart surgery. In some states, certified nurse practitioners work independently within the scope of their training and expertise.

Exercise Physiologists

Many universities offer undergraduate and postgraduate curricula in exercise physiology and performance. Related fields of study include exercise physiology, kinesiology (the physiology of movement), and physical education. The American College of Sports Medicine has developed specific training and performance standards as part of its program to certify clinical professionals involved in exercise and rehabilitation. Individuals trained in these areas are usually not covered by state medical licensure laws. They work under the auspices of a licensed physician when they provide cardiac rehabilitation services.

Athletic Trainers

Athletic trainers complete a college-level curriculum and are certified after passing an examination given by the National Athletic Trainers Association. They are licensed as health professionals in some states. In addition to providing first aid to injured athletes, they work closely with physicians and physical therapists. Athletic trainers directly administer and oversee rehabilitation exercises for injured athletes.

Massage Therapists

Licensed massage therapists provide therapy for strains and sprains. They provide direct relief of pain—not only with therapeutic massage but also by the application of heat, cold, and ultrasound. The quality of training and the licensure requirements for therapeutic massage vary from state to state. A referral from one of the practitioners described above is the best way to ensure the competence of a therapist.

THE TEAM APPROACH TO RECOVERY AND REHABILITATION

Whom you see for help may depend on the type and severity of your problem. It also depends on what point you have reached in your recovery and rehabilitation. Physician involvement is most important and most extensive during your immediate recovery and early rehabilitation process. Once healing and recovery from an injury are under way, the physician's role is reduced, and direct supervision may be delegated to nonphysician exercise professionals. If you are under continuing medical treatment, your physician may serve in an advisory or supervisory role during rehabilitation. The physician remains a vital link in your rehabilitation program.

The team of rehabilitation professionals may be a close-knit one, all practicing under one roof in a sports medicine center. Or it may be a loose confederation of independently functioning professionals. In either case, consider yourself the captain of your rehab team. Take charge of your own outcome by encouraging interaction among all of the professionals who are helping you get back into action. And if these professionals don't communicate with one another (which is sometimes the case), *it's up to you to make sure that you're getting advice that is consistent, compatible, and appropriate for your rehabilitation.* Stay on top of your rehabilitation program, and you'll be back into action with strength, success, and confidence.

Bibliography

Allred, E., E. Bleecker, B. Chaitman, T. Dahms, S. Gottlieb, J. Hackney, M. Pagano, R. Selvester, S. Walden, and J. Warren. "Short-Term Effects of Carbon Monoxide Exposure on the Exercise Performance of Subjects with Coronary Artery Disease." *The New England Journal of Medicine* 321, no. 21 (1989): 1426–1432.

American College of Sports Medicine. "Position Stand—The Prevention of Thermal Injuries During Distance Running." *Medicine and Science in Sports and Exercise* 19, no. 5 (1985): 529–533.

———. "Position Stand—Proper and Improper Weight Loss Programs." *Medicine and Science in Sports and Exercise* 15, no. 1 (1989): ix–xiii.

———. "Position Stand—The Recommended Quantity and Quality of Exercise for Developing and Maintaining Cardiorespiratory and Muscular Fitness in Healthy Adults." *Medicine and Science in Sports and Exercise* 22, no. 2 (1990): 265–271.

Anderson, B., and E. Burke. "Scientific, Medical, and Practical Aspects of Stretching." *Clinics in Sports Medicine* 10, no. 1 (1991): 63–86.

Anthony, J. "Psychologic Aspects of Exercise." *Clinics in Sports Medicine* 10, no. 1 (1991): 171–180.

Aronen, J. "Shoulder Rehabilitation." *Clinics in Sports Medicine* 4, no. 3 (1985): 477–493.

Artal, R., M. Friedman, and J. McNitt-Gray. "Orthopedic Problems in Pregnancy." *The Physician and Sportsmedicine* 18, no. 9 (1990): 93–105.

Askew, E. "Role of Fat Metabolism in Exercise." *Clinics in Sports Medicine* 3, no. 3 (1984): 605–621.

Auerbach, P. "Marine Envenomations." *The New England Journal of Medicine* 325, no. 7 (1991): 486–493.

Berg, R., and J. Cassells, eds. *The Second Fifty Years—Promoting Health and Preventing Disability.* Washington, D.C.: National Academy Press, 1990.

Blair, S., H. Kohn III, R. Paffenbarger, et al. "Physical Fitness and All-Cause Mortality." *The Journal of the American Medical Association* 262, no. 17 (1989): 2395–2401.

Bloom, M. "Differentiating Between Meniscal and Patellar Pain." *The Physician and Sportsmedicine* 17, no. 8 (1989): 95–108.

Blumenthal, M. "Sports-Aggravated Allergies." *The Physician and Sportsmedicine* 18, no. 12 (1990): 52–66.

Brown, M. "Special Considerations During Rehabilitation of the Aged Athlete." *Clinics in Sports Medicine* 8, no. 4 (1989): 893–901.

Burns, T., J. Steadman, and W. Rodkey. "Alpine Skiing and the Mature Athlete." *Clinics in Sports Medicine* 10, no. 2 (1991): 327–342.

Cabrera, J., and F. McCue. "Nonosseous Athletic Injuries of the Elbow, Forearm, and Hand." *Clinics in Sports Medicine* 5, no. 4 (1986): 681–700.

Chow, R., J. Harrison, and C. Notarius. "Effect of Two Randomized Programs on Bone Mass of Healthy Postmenopausal Women." *British Medical Journal* 295 (1987): 1441–1444.

Church, V. "Venom Immunotherapy—When Should You Recommend It?" *The Physician and Sportsmedicine* 19, no. 8 (1990): 118–124.

Clark, N. "Social Drinking and Athletes." *The Physician and Sportsmedicine* 17, no. 10 (1989): 95–100.

Clarkson-Smith, L., and A. Hartley. "Relationships Between Physical Exercise and Cognitive Abilities in Older Adults." *Psychology and Aging* 4, no. 2 (1989): 183–189.

Claytor, R. "Stress Reactivity: Hemodynamic Adjustments in Trained and Untrained Humans." *Medicine and Science in Sports and Exercise* 23, no. 7 (1991): 873–881.

Coats, A. "Guidelines for Physical Training in Patients with Congestive Heart Failure." *Practical Cardiology* 17, no. 9 (1991): 34–40.

Committee on Exercise and Cardiac Rehabilitation of the Council on Clinical Cardiology, American Heart Association (P. McHenry, Chmn). "Statement on Exercise—A Position Statement for Health Professionals." *Circulation* 81, no. 1 (1990): 396–398.

Costill, D. "Water and Electrolyte Requirements During Exercise." *Clinics in Sports Medicine* 3, no. 3 (1984): 639–648.

Costill, D., and E. Fox. "Energetics of Marathon Running." *Medicine and Science in Sports* 1 (1969): 81–86.

Couzens, G. "How to Detect Lyme Disease." *The Physician and Sportsmedicine* 20, no. 4 (1992): 140–147.

Cowart, V. "Should Epileptics Exercise?" *The Physician and Sportsmedicine* 14, no. 9 (1986): 183–191.

Cox, M. "Exercise Training Programs and Cardiorespiratory Adaptation." *Clinics in Sports Medicine* 10, no. 1 (1991): 19–32.

Cress, M., P. Thomas, J. Johnson, F. Kasch, R. Cassens, E. Smith, and J. Agre. "Effect of Training on VO_{2max}, Thigh Strength, and Muscle Morphology in Septuagenarian Women." *Medicine and Science in Sports and Exercise* 23, no. 6 (1991): 752–758.

Davis, A., and Carragee, E. "Sciatica: Treating a Painful Symptom." *The Physician and Sportsmedicine* 20, no. 1 (1992): 126–137.

Derscheid, G., and W. Brown. "Rehabilitation of the Ankle." *Clinics in Sports Medicine* 4, no. 3 (1985): 527–544.

deVries, H. "Tranquilizer Effect of Exercise: A Critical Review." *The Physician and Sportsmedicine* 9, no. 11 (1981): 47–55.

Diamond, S. "Exercise and Headaches." *The Physician and Sportsmedicine* 19, no. 8 (1991): 79–94.

Dickinson, A., and K. Bennett. "Therapeutic Exercise." *Clinics in Sports Medicine* 4, no. 3 (1985): 417–429.

Dishman, R. "Medical Psychology in Exercise and Sport." *Medical Clinics of North America* 69, no. 1 (1985): 123–143.

Dohm, G. "Protein Nutrition for the Athlete." *Clinics in Sports Medicine* 3, no. 3 (1984): 595–604.

Dreyfuss, I. "Athletic Supporters: Comfort and Safety." *The Physician and Sportsmedicine* 18, no. 12 (1990): 116–123.

———. "Desert Shield: Military Wins Battle Against Heat Injury." *The Physician and Sportsmedicine* 19, no. 6 (1991): 141–145.

Duthel, J., J. Vallon, G. Martin, J. Ferret, R. Mathieu, and R. Videman. "Caffeine and Sport: Role of Physical Exercise upon Elimination." *Medicine and Science in Sports and Exercise* 23, no. 8 (1991): 980–985.

Eichner, E. "Circadian Rhythms in Medicine and Sports." *IM Internal Medicine for the Specialist* 11, no. 6 (1990): 58–63.

Eldridge, L., S. Hoecherl, J. Sheridan, et al. "Coronary Heart Disease Attributed to Sedentary Life-Style." *Morbidity and Mortality Weekly Report* 39, no. 32 (1990): 541–544.

Elia, E. "Exercise and the Elderly." *Clinics in Sports Medicine* 10, no. 1 (1991): 141–155.

Ellman, M., R. Neviaser, and R. Willkens. "Shoulder Pain: The Elusive Diagnosis." *Patient Care* 25 (March 15, 1991): 46–66.

Fiatrone, M., E. Marks, N. Ryan, et al. "High-Intensity Strength Training in Nonagenarians: Effects on Skeletal Muscle." *The Journal of the American Medical Association* 263 (1990): 3029–3034.

Fletcher, G., V. Froelicher, H. Hartley, W. Haskell, and M. Pollock. "Exercise Standards—A Statement for Health Professionals from the American Heart Association." *Circulation* 82, no. 6 (1990): 2286–2322.

Fogoros, R. " 'Runner's Trots': Gastrointestinal Disturbances in Runners." *The Journal of the American Medical Association* 243, no. 17 (1980): 1743–1744.

Fox, S., J. Naughton, and P. Gorman. "Physical Activity and Cardiovascular Health: III. The Exercise Prescription—Frequency and Type of Activity." *Modern Concepts in Cardiovascular Disease* 41, no. 6 (1972): 25–30.

Fry, R., A. Morton, and D. Keast. "Acute Intensive Interval Training and T-Lymphocyte Function." *Medicine and Science in Sports and Exercise* 24, no. 3 (1992): 339–345.

Garrett, W. "Muscle Injuries and Inflammation." *Annals of Sports Medicine* 3, no. 2 (1987): 71–72.

Gibbons, L., K. Cooper, B. Meyer, and R. Ellison. "The Acute Cardiac Risks of Strenuous Exercise." *The Journal of the American Medical Association* 244, no. 16 (1980): 1799–1801.

Gollnick, P. "Role of Carbohydrate in Exercise." *Clinics in Sports Medicine* 3, no. 3 (1984): 583–593.

Goodlin, R., and K. Buckley. "Maternal Exercise." *Clinics in Sports Medicine* 3, no. 4 (1984): 881–894.

Gordon, N., and C. Scott. "The Role of Exercise in the Primary and Secondary Prevention of Coronary Artery Disease." *Clinics in Sports Medicine* 10, no. 1 (1991): 87–103.

Green, G. "Gastrointestinal Disorders in the Athlete." *Clinics in Sports Medicine* 11, no. 2 (1992): 453–470.

Grover, R., C. Tucker, S. McGroarty, and R. Travis. "The Coronary Stress of Skiing at High Altitude." *Archives of Internal Medicine* 150, no. 6 (1990): 1205–1208.

Hanson, P., and Zimmerman, S. "Exertional Heatstroke in Novice Runners." *The Journal of the American Medical Association* 242, no. 2 (1979): 154–157.

Hecker, A. "Nutritional Conditioning for Athletic Competition." *Clinics in Sports Medicine* 3, no. 3 (1984): 567–582.

Helmrich, S., D. Ragland, R. Leung, and R. Paffenbarger. "Physical Activity and Reduced Occurrence of Non-Insulin-Dependent Diabetes Mellitus." *The New England Journal of Medicine* 325, no. 3 (1991): 147–152.

Herring, S., and K. Nilson. "Introduction to Overuse Injuries." *Clinics in Sports Medicine* 6, no. 2 (1987): 225–241.

Holloszy, J. "Adaptations of Muscular Tissues to Training." *Progress in Cardiovascular Diseases* 18, no. 6 (1976): 445–458.

Hopkins, M. "Passive Smoking as Determined by Salivary Cotinine and Plasma Carboxyhemoglobin Levels in Adults and School-Aged Children of Smoking and Nonsmoking Parents: Effects on Physical Fitness." *Annals of Sports Medicine* 5, no. 2 (1990): 96–104.

Ike, R., R. Lampman, and C. Castor. "Arthritis and Aerobic Exercise: A Review." *The Physician and Sportsmedicine* 17, no. 2 (1989): 128–140.

Jenkins, D., T. Wolever, V. Vuksan, F. Brighenti, S. Cunnane, A. Rao, A. Jenkins, G. Buckley, R. Patten, W. Singer, P. Corey, and R. Josse. "Nibbling Versus Gorging: Metabolic Advantages of Increased Meal Frequency." *The New England Journal of Medicine* 321, no. 14 (1989): 929–934.

Johnson, R. "Skiing and Snowboarding Injuries." *Postgraduate Medicine* 88, no. 8 (1990): 36–50.

Kannel, W., and R. Abott. "Incidence and Prognosis of Unrecognized Myocardial Infarction. An Update on the Framingham Study." *The New England Journal of Medicine* 311 (1984): 1144–1147.

Kannus, P., and R. Johnson. "Downhill Skiing Injuries: Trends to Watch for This Season." *The Journal of Musculoskeletal Medicine* 8, no. 1 (1991): 13–30.

Kasch, F., J. Boyer, S. Van Camp, L. Verity, and J. Wallace. "The Effect of Physical Activity and Inactivity on Aerobic Power in Older Men (A Longitudinal Study)." *The Physician and Sportsmedicine* 18, no. 4 (1990): 73–83.

Katch, F., and S. Drumm. "Effects of Different Modes of Strength Training on Body Composition and Anthropometry." *Clinics in Sports Medicine* 5, no. 3 (1986): 413–459.

Kaufmann, D. "Protein as an Energy Substrate During Intense Exercise." *Annals of Sports Medicine* 5, no. 3 (1990): 142–143.

Kelemen, M., M. Effron, S. Valenti, and K. Stewert. "Exercise Training Combined with Antihypertensive Therapy." *Journal of the American Medical Association* 263, no. 20 (1990): 2766–2771.

Knight, K. "Guidelines for Rehabilitation of Sports Injuries." *Clinics in Sports Medicine* 4, no. 3 (1985): 405–416.

Knochel, J. "Environmental Heat Illness." *Archives of Internal Medicine* 133, no. 5 (1974): 841–864.

Kovan, J., and D. McKeag. "Lower Extremity Overuse Injuries in Aerobic Dancers." *The Journal of Musculoskeletal Medicine* 9, no. 4 (1992): 43–52.

Kurzweil, P., and D. Jackson. "When Low Back Pain Sidelines Recreational Athletes." *The Journal of Musculoskeletal Medicine* 9, no. 1 (1992): 24–40.

Landry, G., and D. Allen. "Diabetes Mellitus and Exercise." *Clinics in Sports Medicine* 11, no. 2 (1992): 403–418.

Latella, F., W. Conkling, and the Editors of Consumer Reports Books. *Get in Shape, Stay in Shape.* Mount Vernon, N.Y.: Consumers Union, 1989.

Leach, R., and J. Miller. "Lateral and Medial Epicondylitis of the Elbow." *Clinics in Sports Medicine* 6, no. 2 (1987): 259–272.

Leach, R., A. Schepsis, and H. Takai. "Achilles Tendinitis—Don't Let It Be an Athlete's Downfall." *The Physician and Sportsmedicine* 19, no. 8 (1991): 87–92.

Lichtman, S., K. Pisarska, E. Berman, M. Peston, H. Dowling, E. Offenbacher, H. Weisel, S. Heshka, D. Matthews, and S. Heymsfield. "Discrepancy Between Self-Reported and Actual Caloric Intake and Exercise in Obese Subjects." *The New England Journal of Medicine* 327, no. 27 (1992): 1893–1898.

Lorentzen, D., and L. Lawson. "Selected Sports Bras: A Biomechanical Analysis of Breast Motion While Jogging." *The Physician and Sportsmedicine* 15, no. 5 (1987): 128–139.

Lowenthal, D., M. Pollock, and E. Paran. "Age, Drug, and Exercise Interactions in the Treatment of Hypertension." *Annals of Sports Medicine* 5, no. 4 (1990): 181–190.

Mangi, R., P. Jokl, and O. Dayton. *The Runner's Complete Medical Guide.* New York: Summit Books, 1979.

———. *Sports Fitness and Training.* New York: Pantheon Books, 1987.

Manson, J., E. Rimm, M. Stampfer, G. Colditz, W. Willwitt, A. Krolewski, B. Rosner, C. Hennekens, and F. Speizer. "Physical Activity and Incidence of Non-Insulin-Dependent Diabetes Mellitus in Women." *Lancet* 338 (1991): 774–778.

Marcus, R., B. Drinkwater, G. Dalsky, J. Dufek, D. Raab, C. Slemenda, and C. Snow-Harter. "Osteoporosis and Exercise in Women." *Medicine and Science in Sports and Exercise* 24, no. 6 Supplement (1992): S301–S307.

Mattalino, A., J. Deese, and E. Campbell. "Office Evaluation and Treatment of Lower Extremity Injuries in the Runner." *Clinics in Sports Medicine* 8, no. 3 (1989): 461–475.

McCarroll, J., A. Rettig, and K. Shelbourne. "Injuries in the Amateur Golfer." *The Physician and Sportsmedicine* 18, no. 3 (1990): 122–126.

McCarthy, P. "How Much Protein Do Athletes Really Need?" *The Physician and Sportsmedicine* 17, no. 5 (1989): 170–175.

McClennan, J., and J. McClennan. "Cycling and the Older Athlete." *Clinics in Sports Medicine* 10, no. 2 (1991): 291–299.

McGinnis, J. "The Public Health Burden of a Sedentary Life-Style." *Medicine and Science in Sports and Exercise* 24, no. 6 Supplement (1992): S196–S200.

McKeag, D. "The Relationship of Osteoarthritis and Exercise." *Clinics in Sports Medicine* 11, no. 2 (1992): 471–487.

Medical Economics Data. *Physicians' Desk Reference.* Montvale, N.J.: Medical Economics Data, 1993.

Mink, B. "Pulmonary Concerns and the Exercise Prescription." *Clinics in Sports Medicine* 10, no. 1 (1991): 105–116.

Montgomery, L., and P. Deuster. "Acute Antihistamine Ingestion Does Not Affect Muscle Strength and Endurance." *Medicine and Science in Sports and Exercise* 23, no. 9 (1991): 1016–1019.

———. "Ingestion of an Antihistamine Does Not Affect Exercise Performance." *Medicine and Science in Sports and Exercise* 24, no. 3 (1992): 383–388.

Muller, J., and G. Tofler. "Circadian Variation and Cardiovascular Disease." *The New England Journal of Medicine* 323, no. 14 (1991): 1038–1039.

Murray, R., G. Paul, J. Seifert, and D. Eddy. "Responses to Varying Rates of Carbohydrate Ingestion During Exercise." *Medicine and Science in Sports and Exercise* 23, no. 6 (1991): 713–718.

Nadel, E., C. Wenger, M. Roberts, J. Stolwijk, and E. Cafarelli. "Physiologic Defenses Against the Hyperthermia of Exercise." *Annals of the New York Academy of Sciences* 301 (1977): 98–109.

Nygaard, I., J. DeLancey, L. Arnsdorf, and E. Murphy. "Exercise and Incontinence." *Obstetrics and Gynecology* 75, no. 5 (1990): 848–851.

Panza, J., S. Epstein, and A. Quyyumi. "Circadian Variation in Vascular Tone and Its Relation to Alpha-Sympathetic Vasoconstrictor Activity." *The New England Journal of Medicine* 325, no. 14 (1991): 986–990.

Pennington, J. *Bowes & Church's Food Values of Portions Commonly Used.* Philadelphia: J. B. Lippincott Company, 1989.

Pollock, M., and J. Wilmore. *Exercise in Health and Disease.* Philadelphia: W. B. Saunders Company, 1990.

Preventive and Rehabilitative Exercise Committee of the American College of Sports Medicine (R. Pate, Ph.D., Chair). *Guidelines for Exercise Testing and Prescription.* 4th ed. Philadelphia: Lee & Febiger, 1991.

Prince, R., M. Smith, I. Dick, R. Price, P. Webb, N. Henderson, and M. Harris. "Prevention of Postmenopausal Osteoporosis—A Comparative Study of Exercise, Calcium Supplementation, and Hormone-Replacement Therapy." *The New England Journal of Medicine* 325, no. 17 (1991): 1189–1195.

Quadagno, D., L. Faquin, G. Lim, W. Kuminka, and R. Moffatt. "The Menstrual Cycle: Does It Affect Athletic Performance?" *The Physician and Sportsmedicine* 19, no. 3 (1991): 121–124.

Radack, K., and R. Wyderski. "Conservative Management of Intermittent Claudication." *Annals of Internal Medicine* 113, no. 2 (1990): 135–146.

Ramotar, J. "Royalty or Commoner: Horses Don't Discriminate." *The Physician and Sportsmedicine* 18, no. 9 (1990): 40–41.

Reichel, M., and D. Laub. "From Acne to Black Heel: Common Skin Injuries in Sports." *The Physician and Sportsmedicine* 20, no. 2 (1992): 111–118.

Richardson, A., and J. Miller. "Swimming and the Older Athlete." *Clinics in Sports Medicine* 10, no. 2 (1991): 301–316.

Rigsby, L., R. Dishman, A. Jackson, G. Maclean, and P. Raven. "Effects of Exercise Training on Men Seropositive for the Human Immunodeficiency Virus-1." *Medicine and Science in Sports and Exercise* 24, no. 1 (1992): 6–12.

Rosenbloom, D., and J. Sutton. "Drugs and Exercise." *Medical Clinics of North America* 69, no. 1 (1985): 177–187.

Roy, S., and R. Irvin. *Sports Medicine—Prevention, Evaluation, Management, and Rehabilitation.* Englewood Cliffs, N.J.: Prentice-Hall, 1983.

Sacks, J., P. Holmgreen, S. Smith, and D. Sosin. "Bicycle-Associated Head Injuries and Deaths in the United States from 1984 through 1988." *The Journal of the American Medical Association* 266, no. 21 (1991): 3016–3018.

Samples, P. "Experts: Don't Swim with Soft Contacts In." *The Physician and Sportsmedicine* 17, no. 9 (1989): 34–36.

Sayce, V., and I. Fraser. *Exercise for Arthritis.* Mount Vernon, N.Y.: Consumer Reports Books, 1989.

Sazy, J., and H. Horstmann. "Exercise Participation After Menopause." *Clinics in Sports Medicine* 10, no. 2 (1991): 359–369.

Schelkun, P. "Exercise and Breast-Feeding Mothers." *The Physician and Sportsmedicine* 19, no. 4 (1991): 109–116.

Schon, L., D. Baxter, and T. Clanton. "Chronic Exercise-Induced Leg Pain in Active People—More Than Just Shin Splints." *The Physician and Sportsmedicine* 20, no. 1 (1992): 100–114.

Sehnert, K. *How to Be Your Own Doctor—Sometimes.* New York: Grosset & Dunlap, 1975.

Shangold, M. "Gynecologic Concerns in the Woman Athlete." *Clinics in Sports Medicine* 3, no. 4 (1984): 869–879.

Sheps, D., M. Herbst, A. Hinderliter, K. Adams, L. Ekelund, J. O'Neil, G. Goldstein, P. Bromberg, J. Dalton, M. Ballenger, S. Davis, and G. Kock. "Production of Arrhythmias by Elevated Carboxyhemoglobin in Patients with Coronary Artery Disease." *Annals of Internal Medicine* 113, no. 5 (1990): 343–351.

Sherman, W., and A. Albright. "Exercise and Type I Diabetes." *Sports Science Exchange* 3, no. 25 (1990): 1–6.

———. "Exercise and Type II Diabetes." *Sports Science Exchange* 4, no. 37 (1992).

Siscovick, D., N. Weiss, R. Fletcher, and T. Lasky. "The Incidence of Primary Cardiac Arrest During Vigorous Exercise." *The New England Journal of Medicine* 311, no. 14 (1984): 874–877.

Spencer, G. "Projections of the Population of the United States by Age, Sex, and Race: 1988 to 2080." *Current Population Reports Series*. P-25, no. 1018. Washington, D.C.: U.S. Bureau of the Census, January 1989.

Stamler, R., J. Stanler, F. Gosch, J. Civinelli, J. Fishman, P. McKeever, A. McDonald, and A. Dyer. "Primary Prevention of Hypertension by Nutritional-Hygienic Means." *The Journal of the American Medical Association* 262, no. 13 (1989): 1801–1807.

Stone, M., and G. Wilson. "Resistive Training and Selected Effects." *The Medical Clinics of North America* 69, no. 1 (1985): 109–122.

Tanji, J. "Exercise and the Hypertensive Athlete." *Clinics in Sports Medicine* 11, no. 2 (1992): 291–302.

Teitz, C., and D. Cook. "Rehabilitation of Neck and Low Back Injuries." *Clinics in Sports Medicine* 4, no. 3 (1985): 455–476.

Thomas, R. "Caffeine and Arrhythmias: What Are the Risks?" *Your Patient & Fitness* 5, no. 5 (1991): 6–8.

Thornton, J. "Carboloading and Endurance: A New Look." *The Physician and Sportsmedicine* 17, no. 10 (1989): 149–156.

———. "Common Concerns About the Common Cold." *The Physician and Sportsmedicine* 18, no. 6 (1990): 120–126.

Ting, A. "Running and the Older Athlete." *Clinics in Sports Medicine* 10, no. 2 (1991): 319–325.

Van Camp, S., and R. Peterson. "Cardiovascular Complications of Outpatient Cardiac Rehabilitation Programs." *The Journal of the American Medical Association* 256, no. 9 (1986): 1160–1163.

Vander, L., B. Franklin, and M. Rubenfire. "Cardiovascular Complications of Recreational Activity." *The Physician and Sportsmedicine* 10, no. 1 (1982): 89–97.

Van Duser, B., and P. Raven. "The Effects of Oral Smokeless Tobacco on the Cardiorespiratory Response to Exercise." *Medicine and Science in Sports and Exercise* 24, no. 3 (1992): 389–394.

Vereschagin, K., W. Firtch, L. Caputo, and M. Hoffman. "Transient Paresthesia in Stair-Climber's Feet." *The Physician and Sportsmedicine* 21, no. 2 (1993): 63–69.

Viitasalo, M., R. Kala, A. Eisalo, and P. Halonen. "Ventricular Arrhythmias During Exercise Testing, Jogging, and Sedentary Life." *Chest* 71, no. 1 (1979): 21–26.

Wasserman, K., and B. Whipp. "Exercise Physiology in Health and Disease." *American Review of Respiratory Disease* 112 (1975): 219–249.

Weil, R. "Weight Training and Diabetes Mellitus." *Practical Diabetology* 9, no. 3 (1990): 20–23.

Weinstein, S., and S. Herring. "Nerve Problems and Compartment Syndromes in the Hand, Wrist, and Forearm." *Clinics in Sports Medicine* 11, no. 1 (1992): 161–188.

Wheeler, K. "Sports Nutrition for the Primary Care Physician: The Importance of Carbohydrate." *The Physician and Sportsmedicine* 17, no. 5 (1989): 106–117.

Wilmore, J. "The Aging of Bone and Muscle." *Clinics in Sports Medicine* 10, no. 2 (1991): 231–244.

Index